HUGS

FROM THE

REFRIGERATOR

HUGS

FROM THE

REFRIGERATOR

James McClernan, Ed.D.

Westport Publishers, Inc.
Kansas City, Missouri

Printed in the United States of America

Library of Congress Cataloging-in-Publication Data

McClernan, James 1935-
    Hugs from the refrigerator / by James McClernan, Ed.D.
    p.   cm.
    Includes bibliographical references.
    ISBN 0-933701-61-6
    1. Reducing.   I. title.
RM222.2.M4334   1993
613.2'5--dc20   93-24657
                                                       CIP

TABLE OF CONTENTS

Foreword

During the 1930s, the average American expended approximately 2,400 calories in activity each day. By the 1990s, that figure had dropped to a mere 600 to 800 calories. Obviously, as technology increases, the population's activity level decreases. Just glance back over the past 10 to 15 years. Push mowers evolved into tractors. The Saturday morning car scrubbing has become a trip to the automatic car wash. Manual laundry developed into a fully automated system. Even clerical workers soon found that they burned fewer calories after switching from a typewriter to a desktop computer, by gaining up to seven pounds!

Although Americans are eating fewer calories today than at the turn of the century, and the availability of healthy food has never been so prevalent, obesity is almost at epidemic proportions. Rapidly advancing technology has assisted in the increasing of the population's sedentary levels. But to counteract these negative results, science has also accomplished major discoveries in the domain of personal health.

Research is continually acknowledging the slow evolutionary process at which the human body has been consistently adapting itself to its environment over millions of years. For example, in relation to weight loss, for thousands of generations the number one nutrition-related cause of death was starvation. (And it still is today in many parts of the world.) The human body has become naturally self-adjusting. These automatic adjustments are easily experienced by everyone in feelings of hunger; in the desire for calorie-rich foods (including simple sugars and fats); in the ease of gaining extra storage of calories even when food is in abundance; in the body's continual resistance to utilizing fat as energy (thus making fat loss difficult); and in the speed at which the body replaces the lost fat from starvation (dieting) methods.

Oddly enough, very few weight-loss methods acknowledge this fact and then insist that the answer to success lies in trying to *trick* that intricate network of organic signals that we've inherited from millions of years of evolutionary development. This cannot be done! And the participants of the majority of weight-loss programs are now learning this after much frustration.

At the Cooper Aerobics Center, we view preventative medicine and healthful exercise, along with proper nutrition, as the best approaches to good health. Just as we should avail ourselves of as much "opportunistic exercise" as possible, so should we aim at developing healthful eating habits. The solution for long-term weight control is making sure that the strategies used coincide with the body's biology and don't work against it. Therefore, for a successful fat-reduction regimen, a long-term, objective view must be adopted. What we must avoid is the perspective that benefits only the popular commercial programs, those that insist on nursing the public's emotional whim to lose fat quickly, no matter the cost to the participant.

Hugs from the Refrigerator is one of the few books I have read that integrates all the complicated physiological and psychological concerns from an objective, scientific viewpoint. *Hugs from the Refrigerator* repudiates the quick weight-loss mentality and provides the reader with the tools to recapture personal responsibility for his or her own health.

It is not incongruous that only one in five Americans actually works hard enough at significant personal preventative health measures to substantially affect his or her life. Four out of five Americans want a national health care policy that will guarantee medical services for all. I begin to wonder if these people are divided into two groups whose ideas are either, "It is my responsibility to do all I can to ensure my future health," or "I can live my life by mere whim, evading my negative health practices because the government will take care of me when I get sick."

The annual health care bill is fast approaching $1 trillion and draining the economy. A majority seems to be screaming, "We need a new system now!" Some believe that this new system should be the government's obligation. However, the objective reality is that the onus of the primary responsibility of our own personal health is on each and every one of us, individually!

As a reader of *Hugs from the Refrigerator*, you are in a select group that is taking the initiative and the responsibility for your health. Maybe this is your first preventative book. Maybe you are searching for the much-needed genuine education that will enhance your present personal lifestyle. If so, I sincerely welcome you. And above all, I believe this is the finest start you could obtain toward beginning your healthy future.

Philip Walker, M.S.
Fitness Management Consultant
The Cooper Aerobics Center

ACKNOWLEDGMENTS

This book is the result of many influences. Among those who have directly and indirectly helped me develop my philosophy of self-directed weight loss through wellness are Albert Ellis, author and director of the Institute for Rational-Emotive Therapy; Nathaniel Branden, author and director of the Branden Institute for Self-Esteem; George Leonard, former editor of *Look* and author of *Mastery*; Deepak Chopra, with the Center for Longevity and Human Potential; The Cooper Aerobics Center; the Association for Humanistic Psychology; and the Institute of Noetic Sciences.

INTRODUCTION

Paving the Road to Hell
With Good Intentions

The faces look full of hope, insight, and understanding after completing a six-hour workshop. I feel stimulated and self-satisfied. I held the audience's attention and the message appeared to have gotten through. I talked about the futility of weight-loss diets, the importance of risk-taking to long-term change, going from external to internal motivation, getting beyond procrastination, letting go of the quest for magical answers as the first step to long-term success, etc.

Then someone bursts my balloon with a question that lets me know the point has been missed. This has been played out many times. The questions I find so devastating usually go something like "How many calories are there in your diet?" or the classic "Do I have to exercise before I lose enough weight to look good in my exercise outfit?" What they let me know is that they still count on me, the program, or the product to change them — that changing self-doubt isn't their goal. Coming to the weight-loss group and following the plan are okay, but working on underlying causes and risking change are difficult and frightening, and that is when the whole weight-loss-through-wellness scheme breaks down.

It is not with pride that I have learned of my own part in the Great American Fat Rip-Off. Having a family history of obesity problems and being sensitive to people with this problem, it was always my intention to help. But in my drive to do that, at times I had served the weight-loss *industry* better than those who use it.

I first became involved by designing and conducting research for a hospital that was already treating alcoholism and smoking. One treatment the hospital used was aversion conditioning, which pairs a negative experience (physical, non-harmful pain) with an old pleasurable experience (eating fattening foods) to create a subconscious aversion to the formerly pleasurable experience. I quickly found that aversion conditioning didn't work.

I did, however, learn a great deal from using it. First, I saw the power of offering what appeared to be *magic*. With a small two-paragraph announcement about the research and my need for subjects in a small suburban newspaper, I received 500 phone calls the first week.

Second, I learned that once those in the aversion conditioning group realized the magic was far less powerful than their desire to eat, they were ready to consider conventional methods, such as gradual self-change.

Third, the hospital told me the high treatment cost was a part of why clients quit smoking or drinking. For a while I assumed that was correct and that it would apply to the weight-loss program as well. But only recently, when I've reviewed long-term success rates for all commercial programs, does it appear that paying for help may actually *reduce* chances for long-term success. I've found that the more people pay for help, the higher their expectations for the program to change them and the less they seek *intrinsic* change. In fact, members of my groups who weren't charged the fee actually did better than those who pay for commercial programs today.

I also learned that when aversion conditioning was paired with imagery, changes lasted longer, though they were still temporary. When I used imagery alone, I found it was more powerful than the aversion conditioning.

Aversion conditioning was the least effective method I tried. Two methods that were more effective were the comprehensive wellness group, which didn't excite the volunteers because it focused on health and was slow, and the existential discussion group, which dealt with each member's freedom to make choices.

The existential group did as well or better than the other groups. They discussed why it is impossible to escape free choice when we are aware of choices. There were no discussions about weight loss, diet, exercise, hypnosis, or anything like that. In fact, other than weighing in to qualify and weighing at the end of the program, nothing could be seen as treatment for weight loss. Most likely, the success of these people came from their realization that any change was up to them.

This should have been my biggest clue that expensive, full-service programs would never be effective for large numbers of people. **The more that people look to others for change in their own behavior, the less they seek change within themselves.**

Finally, the research showed that the value of the weight-loss support group faded in a few months. First I thought that just switching to another group was the answer. Then I believed that switching groups was what many do to renew the initial value of a group. Now I understand that different people change at different rates, and some may actually use group to avoid change.

After my experience with aversion conditioning, I ran my own wellness weight-loss programs both in and out of the hospital. The weight-loss-through-wellness program sold much better in a hospital setting, probably because of the authority we tend to place in the medical community. Unfortunately, a weight-loss-through-wellness program would never make the hospital large profits. So it was never promoted.

I was also involved briefly with another hospital that was doing gastroplasty (stomach stapling) and liposuction (surgical removal of fat cells). I was asked in because they had no trained counselors, which they had advertised as part of their program. I was told I could work with the patients on an individual basis and run weekly group meetings. However, I could only see the patients *after* the operation. It was quickly apparent that the surgeons did not want me to talk anybody out of surgery for social or emotional reasons.

Two sessions with these patients convinced me that some were not only seriously disturbed, but they were also angry with the misinformation and omission of information prior to signing up for the operation, not to mention the $15,000 they had paid for their unhappiness. They had *not* been told that their desire to eat would be just as great after the surgery; that the majority would regain all their weight loss plus more; or that their stapled stomach could stretch to accommodate larger amounts of food. Nor were they warned of the pain from the foot-long incision or how many times they would regurgitate their food. And they weren't told they could have many of the same nutritional problems as a person on a partial fast.

Just before I was about to give up on hospital-based programs, my resolve weakened and I joined in with the newest weight-loss fad: a medically supervised liquid fast that promised big money for the hospital and rapid weight loss for the participants.

Such radical programs usually die of their own weight because of their extremely poor long-term success rate; however, those determined to have the "quick-fix" may attempt a second and third try, blaming themselves before deciding the program doesn't work. I believed, incorrectly, that the clients would realize this at least as soon as those in the aversion program had. But fasting did provide the quick weight loss from water, muscle, and fat, so the reality of fasting came more slowly.

The fasting program started about the time Oprah Winfrey made her announcement that she had lost 67 pounds on a liquid fast. Business was overwhelming. For the first year we were always behind the demand.

From the start there were deficiencies. There was, in my opinion, inadequate training for the doctors and counselors. The dietitians, who came from the hospital staff, added this work to their regular duties. It was clear from private conversations that they did not believe fasting was in the best interest of the patients. Finally, the nurses on our staff were selected not because of any special training in weight problems but because they were overweight. They could serve as role models. (Both nurses lost large amounts of weight, yet they fell into the typical pattern. Even with the insight, support, and high-profile position in the group, they were soon on their way back up the weight scale. Disenchanted, depressed, angry, and embarrassed, they resigned.)

This program was the worst I had been involved with, if for no other reason than that its long-term ineffectiveness was disguised by its professional cover as a hospital-based, physician-supervised program.

The terms "client" and "patient" being used together is one example of how the philosophy of hospital-based programs makes long-term change unlikely. A "patient" is someone who is ill or injured and who must passively wait for recovery or seek treatment. Fat, in and of itself, is only a potential precursor to illness. Calling the clients "patients" implies that a medical treatment is available and necessary to cure fat. The patient need only be passively compliant and, *voilà*, the fat will be gone; he or she will be "cured."

The whole program was part of a Great American Fat Rip-Off, an expensive facade, run by professionals in a trusted hospital setting. Add to this an overweight population with $3,000 worth of expectations, low self-esteem, and fear of rejection — in a society obsessed to meet impossible standards of thinness — and you have a formula for a popular and profitable fat rip-off.

Emotion plays a powerful role. You can see this from the broad spectrum of consumers. Rich and poor, young and old, black and white, doctors, counselors, nurses, engineers, CPAs, teachers, business executives, lawyers

— bright, well-educated people with access to all the information they need to make the sound decision not to enter programs of this type — would join. They shared the belief that if they could just get the weight off *one more time*, they would keep it off for sure.

Believing that the fat somehow kept them from changing their behavior, they concluded that once the fat was gone, they would be in "control." But this was backward. Instead, by changing belief *first*, people seeking weight loss can reach their goals. This is self-efficacy.

Yet after 20 years of trying to nurture self-efficacy using every means known to me, some that I'm not very proud of, I have come to this realization. The more comprehensive and structured the program, the more it costs, the more charismatic the leader, the more gimmicks and products used, and the longer the participants stay with the program, the less likely meaningful, long-term intrinsic change will come about and/or the less likely long-term weight loss will occur. Yet it seems a contradiction to tell people in commercial weight-loss programs not to look outside themselves but rather within themselves for answers. After all, they've paid $3,000, have a respected professional guiding them, and a bunch of other people around them looking for the same magic answer, and they are experiencing it all in a facility devoted to "curing illness."

Then why did I write this book? Is it just another means to encourage people to seek the magic?

No, this book has no magic; it explores finding the magic *inside yourself*. This book is written for those individuals who want to find a direction where, if they will look, work, and take risks, they can bring about not only a healthful weight balance but also a confident sense of harmony along with it. A book won't change you or the belief you have in yourself, but it will give you information about how you can bring about your own change when you are ready.

James McClernan, Ed.D.

CHAPTER 1

Why Me?

When Louise would make her tenth trip to the refrigerator during an evening at home, she usually wasn't thinking, "I'm feeling stressed and I'm going to have a little snack to help me feel better for a few minutes." She initiated each trip in a more mechanical, non-thinking manner. At times, she would notice her frustration as she stood with the refrigerator door open, looking for the vague something that wasn't there twenty minutes ago, still wondering what it could be.

Louise is an actual person. And like millions of other people who do the same thing each day, Louise was bored (anxious), waiting for something to happen to stimulate her when she had no clear direction. It needed to be something that would bring purpose, value, pleasure, excitement, joy, or peace to her life. With Louise, it could just as easily have been anger, fear, sadness, sexual tension, loneliness, or the lack of loving intimacy in her life that inspired those snack trips. But her journey started long before.

As a young girl, Louise would watch from outside the screen door, fearful that her drunk father would hit her mother again. She watched as her father knocked her mother to the floor. Louise was torn with emotions. She felt overwhelmed by guilt, that somehow this was all her fault, that she should be helping her mother. But she was afraid that her dad would leave for good if she tried to help her mother and that both of them would leave her if she couldn't make things better at home.

Would it surprise you to learn that both parents were perfectionists, manifesting feelings of shame and guilt by being critical and demanding of their children? This particularly affected Louise, who, with her lack of self-esteem and feelings of guilt, was a vulnerable target.

She was the baby. Always in the way. She was the one her older sister used to blame for having to stay home to cook and clean instead of having fun with her friends. Louise's mother worked long and hard to support the family, but she was always mad and yelling at her dad. Louise's father responded by getting drunk, gambling, running around with other women, and beating her mother. Louise was sure it was all her fault and wouldn't have blamed her sister or parents if they wanted to leave her. The only thing she could do was to be as good and as helpful and as non-demanding as possible, with the hope that then her family wouldn't want to leave her.

Louise promised herself that she would never show anger like her dad and that she would always work hard like her mother. She could make people laugh. She knew that she could keep her sister happy — and even get to go places with her occasionally — if she asked for nothing and did some of her sister's chores. Yet her mother was critical and demanding, leaving Louise feeling that she could never quite please her no matter how hard she tried.

A deeply felt fear had been instilled in Louise. This fear kept her anxious and on guard for more than 20 years. It was an ongoing fear that she would never be quite good enough and that she must always put others above herself. She believed that she must learn what pleased others and felt guilt if she couldn't please them. Louise's entire life experience had left her ill-prepared to get to know or nurture

herself or to believe in her worth. Instead, she became a perfectionist, too.

All of the time Louise was growing up, the people she depended on the most were models of a behavior that crushed her belief in herself and taught her how to be the consummate people pleaser. She learned to stuff her anger with the only thing that comforted her: a *Hug from the Refrigerator*. With the refrigerator supplying all of her hugs, Louise was about 20 pounds overweight by the time she was twelve. She was shy and quiet, but, of course, well-liked because she was funny, selfless, and appeared to be happy.

Other heavy people may grow up in very different circumstances from those of Louise, with parents who are educated, who don't drink or gamble, who do not physically or emotionally abuse them, and who are supportive of their activities. But they may show subtle, underlying expectations that winning is what approval is all about. It appears as though their performance defines their worth. Thus they become perfectionists.

From the following self-evaluation questionnaire, you can easily see the psychodynamics of how you might have developed into a person who is apt to be compulsive, overweight, and suffering from low self-esteem, ongoing anxiety, and perfectionism to the point of diminishing returns. All you have to do is go through six steps and pick out those aspects of your developmental years that led to what seems to be an uncontrollable, chronic weight problem today.

Development of the Overweight Personality

As you study each of the six steps, reflect on those years from childhood through the present. Then ask yourself and other family members if any of these conditions existed to the extent that they would lead to the behavior described in Step 6. Check those items that seem to apply to your own life.

If one or more of the conditions existed for you in each stage, they likely led to one or more of the conditions in the next stage.

1. ROOT CAUSES: These are factors over which you had little or no control that may have influenced your tendency to be overweight.
   ☐ Genetic predisposition, culture, and family customs.
   ☐ Limited or qualified praise from parents and significant others.
   ☐ High expectations of your parents for you or others.
   ☐ Perfectionistic, obese, alcoholic, indifferent, or absent parent or parents.
   ☐ Overprotective or domineering parent or parents.
   ☐ Role models of high achiever older sibling(s).
   ☐ Verbal, physical, or sexual abuse by adults.
   ☐ Family handicaps: social, emotional, physical, financial, or educational.
   ☐ Environmental conditioning pertaining to eating habits and a negative self-concept.
   ☐ Shortage of information or concern about healthful eating and exercise.
2. THOUGHT PATTERNS: Root causes can affect the nature of your thinking.
   ☐ Disordered thinking (hard to complete thoughts).
   ☐ Poor self-awareness (unaware of how your mind affects your behavior).
   ☐ Narrow perspective (limited view of life and the world).
   ☐ Critical or negative thinking.
   ☐ Closed mind or frightened or angered by new ideas.
   ☐ Defensive; avoiding challenges.
   ☐ High expectations of self and others.
   ☐ Parent message (shoulds, musts, have to be the best).
   ☐ Oversimplifying or catastrophizing life experiences.

☐ Indecision (insecurity and conflict about what is "right").

☐ External focus; what do *they* want? (more attention to others than self).

☐ Denial or suppression of life's realities.

☐ Achievement oriented (if you achieve enough, problems will dissolve).

3. DOMINANT RESULTING EMOTIONS: How and what you think will affect your emotional state.

☐ Fear of failure, rejection, or being unloved.

☐ Guilt about what you do or don't do.

☐ Anxiety or impatience, often without awareness or acknowledgment.

☐ Frustration and contained anger.

☐ Hurt, disappointment, and hypersensitivity.

☐ Loneliness, depression, and low energy.

☐ Manic (exaggerated short-term happiness) or relief.

4. SELF-CONCEPT DEVELOPMENT: Your emotional state in turn determines how you value yourself.

☐ Low self-worth, esteem, and/or trust.

☐ Feelings of inadequacy and dependence.

☐ Helplessness, hopelessness.

☐ Feeling valued only as an achiever.

5. BASIC MOTIVATIONS: Your self-value will affect what motives control your choices and actions.

☐ Affiliation (closely associated in a dependent or subordinate way).

☐ Achievement (to acquire affiliation and "safety from rejection").

☐ Power (to control people and circumstances to be perfect).

6. BEHAVIOR PATTERNS: One or more factors in the five preceding steps will affect how you react in life situations.

☐ Compulsive, need for structure, or focus on detail.

☐ Passive compliance.

□ Procrastination and/or avoidance.

□ Perfectionistic in thinking and behavior.

□ People pleasing with other than family members.

□ Critical, nagging, and accusing with self and family.

□ Controlling, pushy, or manipulative.

□ Hyperactive or sedentary.

□ Difficulty in accepting change.

□ Difficulty in letting go of people, ideas, and possessions.

□ Easily conditioned by external circumstances and events.

□ Neglectful of self to win approval of others

While the family is ultimately important in the development of a chronic weight problem, other factors must also be considered. The family unit is, after all, part of a much larger environment that constantly lets us know what is expected of us and what we must be and do to be accepted and rewarded. In short, it tells us all the things most people want and are willing to work and perform for, the standards we are told to achieve and live by.

We live in a dangerous, competitive world that becomes more so each day. The pace and the influence of our environment, by themselves, can almost assure us that we will spend much of our time with an external focus so we won't be swept away in the current. They also assure that we will have little time to know or understand ourselves and that we must be on guard most of the time so we will lose as seldom as possible. And to the overweight person with low self-esteem, losing is the fear. To lose is to face the ultimate fear of rejection or the withholding of a reward.

With the prospects of being swept away, with losing and rejection always hanging over everyone's heads, the person who has been taught at home not to trust, believe in, or like him or herself is going to be much more anxious and will try much harder to be perfect or to avoid as many challenges as possible. Under these kinds of everyday conditions, stress becomes an often subconscious way of life. Because food is sensually comforting, and taste and aroma create neurochemical reactions in the brain that lead to pleasurable feelings, food can easily become the drug of choice to calm oneself. Of course, when stress is ongoing, a great deal of sensual comforting is desired.

Many of us grew up with a shortage of information about food and exercise. Even now, science is only starting to understand the effects of food on our physical and emotional well-being. To stay abreast of the new research findings and evaluate the disagreements about those findings seems to require a Ph.D. in the field, not to mention an abundance of time to study the information. But this idea is a myth. Those individuals who have been long-term successful on their own found the necessary information they needed very easy to access.

Our culture continues to give us many destructive messages about food, e.g., steak and apple pie are the American way and remember to clean your plate. Not only are many of our conditioning messages destructive, they are also conflicting. The media bombard us with the message that trim is in, then promote all kinds of appealing, high-calorie, non-nutritious foods. We're also encouraged to strive to be the best, the richest, the most beautiful, the happiest. But if you aren't able to achieve those goals while remaining stress-free, you may die prematurely, or at least you won't enjoy your success. And if you do manage to out-perform too many people, you'll probably feel guilty and push yourself even harder to give a great deal back to those whom you've worked so hard to outpace.

With all the straining, conflicts, confusion, guilt, and shame about what we aren't and should be driving us to be compulsive, we long for sensual comforting. Resisting it is more than having the proper information and overcoming genetic predisposition and cultural conditioning. It's more than simply eating fewer calories and burning more.

Louise was taught to be a perfectionist, and when she became aware of the relationship between straining to be perfect and her weight, she was faced with doing many things to bring about self-change. She had to determine what type of perfectionist she was, to what extent her perfectionism related to her weight problem, and how to go about modifying her perfectionist traits.

Louise had a lot to learn about the relationship between fat and perfectionism, about her willingness to take necessary risks, and about her power to change her attitudes and behavior.

This book will lead you on that journey.

CHAPTER 2

The Great American Fat Rip-Off

Americans spend \$33 billion every year trying to lose weight. A 1990 survey by the U.S. government indicates 1/2 of all American women and 1/4 of all American men are on a diet at any given moment. We buy diet pills, exercise equipment, liquid diets, packaged foods, and diet books. We join weight-loss groups, exercise centers, and hospital-sponsored weight-loss programs. We submit to hypnosis and liposuction; we have our stomachs stapled and our jaws wired. Most of us who try one or more of these weight-loss methods either fail to lose any significant amount of weight or we regain it quickly.

Facts on Long-Term Success
And Safety of Diet Programs and Products

The large commercial weight-loss providers publish little or no follow-up studies of a long-term nature. The November 24, 1992, issue of *The New York Times* reports that the leading commercial weight-loss programs offer no reliable information about their success rates. In October of 1993, the Federal Trade Commission took this a step further, charging five of the biggest diet programs with engaging in deceptive advertising. According to the FTC, the companies charged have made unsubstantiated weight-loss claims and used consumer testimonials without showing that they represent typical experiences of dieters in their programs. The FTC has instructed the companies to temper their stories of extraordinary diet successes with disclosures about average success rates or with statements that they are not typical. As of this writing, three of the companies charged have agreed to comply with changes called for by the FTC.

Some commercial programs are good at casting the blame for failure on the individual, claiming that "people are not norms" (that is, statistics don't determine individual behavior) or that unsuccessful customers "did not follow the program as instructed." Additionally, because old programs and products peter out and new ones are born almost monthly, many companies evade the question of documented long-term successes by simply stating that "it is too soon to tell." And, of course, many consumers are eager to believe in the possibility of success, so most are unlikely to press the issue any further.

Of one thing you can be absolutely sure: if any weight-loss method should be proven through independent, sound, indisputable, reproducible research to be safe and long-term effective for large numbers of people, you will read about it in the headlines.

However, the fact is that even though a great deal of sound and independent research on obesity — with a current annual price tag of $500 million — has been conducted on an ongoing basis for the past forty years, little is known about the short- or long-term safety and effectiveness of most of the weight-loss products and methods in use today. At this point, *no* known program, plan, treatment, or product offers long-term effectiveness to other than a very small percentage of individuals. Because a certain number of individuals are going to be successful no matter which means or method they choose to lose weight, it is very possible that the program or treatment involved cannot claim responsibility for even these few successes.

Here are just a few examples of the mass of research literature and regulator scrutiny that give more than sufficient cause to exercise caution before using any commercial program, product, or treatment for weight loss:

- A survey of 95,000 subscribers by *Consumer Reports* magazine found no evidence that commercial weight-loss programs help most people. Their conclusion: you'll probably do best to try reducing on your own. (*Consumer Reports*, June 1993)
- A survey of participants of a pre-packaged food plan who elected to have their pictures and testimonials used in advertisements found that after only 20 months, nearly three-fourths had regained their weight. (*Journal of the American Dietetic Association,* 1989)
- An eight-year experience with a very low-calorie formula diet for control of major obesity, with multidisciplinary group counseling, found a quarter of the patients were unable to adapt to this approach, dropping out within the first three weeks, with only 5% to 10% maintaining weight loss after 18 months. (*International Journal of Obesity*, 1987)
- A San Diego State University analysis of a very low-calorie diet plus behavior modification revealed that fewer than half of a group of 400 dieters completed the program. Those who did complete it regained 70% to 100% of the lost weight within 30 months. (*American Health Magazine*, March 1989)
- In October 1990, Dr. Philip A. Kern, Cedars-Sinai Medical Center in Los Angeles, stated his research indicated that rapid weight loss doubled the activity of the fat-metabolizing enzyme LPL, meaning a certain regain of lost weight after very low-calorie diets.
- At a meeting of the American Heart Association, Dr. Kelly Brownell of Yale University reported that

recent studies show that rapid losses of large amounts of weight create a greater risk of heart attack than keeping a level weight. (*The Arizona Republic*, January 17, 1993)

The list of newspaper and magazine citations exposing the weight-loss industry in America could go on for pages. Many additional articles are in the bibliography.

Congress Checks Truth and Safety

I've listed only a small sample from the research literature available today. In addition, recent Congressional investigations pointed out the need for more rigorous enforcement of truth-in-advertising regulations by the FTC.

These hearings took place in the spring of 1990 under the chairmanship of Representative Ron Wyden from Oregon, heading the House Subcommittee on Regulation, Business Opportunities, and Energy Dealing with Health, Safety, and Consumer Protection Issues Involving Weight-Loss Programs.

The Committee's findings point out not only the physical damage, economic loss, and extremely poor effectiveness of weight-loss programs in the long term but also the undermining of self-efficacy for the consumer.

A few of the excerpts from the important Congressional findings are:

- Sixty percent of medical school graduates don't get adequate training in nutrition, leaving some without even a basic understanding of the complicated physiological and psychological factors in obesity, according to the Association of American Medical Colleges. Nutri/System CEO A. Donald McCulloch admitted his nutrition specialists and behavior counselors get just one week of company training. Dr. Jerry Sutkamp, Medical Director of Physicians Weight Loss Centers, stated, "Our physicians have no special training in nutrition other than what they receive in medical school."
- Liquid diet manufacturers aggressively market their wares to doctors. A sample come-on sug-

gests that a physician can net more than $22,000 yearly treating only 20 patients and more than $70,000 by treating 100.

- According to the Surgeon General's Report on Health and Nutrition, the causes of obesity are poorly understood, and, therefore, knowledge about how to prevent and treat it is also limited.
- State medical boards testified before the subcommittee that their state attorneys general told them *not* to police weight-loss ads because they would be sued by the Federal Trade Commission for restraint of trade. While the FTC has focused on print advertising, it has ignored radio and TV advertising, which many of the biggest plans use exclusively to sell their products.

A public misconception is that if these programs were dangerous, the government would stop them. The Food and Drug Administration is sitting on the sidelines. Nearly 20 years ago the FDA began drafting regulations on over-the-counter weight-loss products. In 1982 the resulting monograph was finally published. Eight years later, that monograph still rested, unimplemented, in the bowels of the FDA's bureaucracy.

Commercial weight-loss programs do not exist in a vacuum. They are skillfully and deliberately exploiting a situation where cultural norms are dramatically out of sync with biological reality. Sudden deaths still occur. The fact that we have not heard about them until recently reflects our lack of any type of tracking mechanism. We have no way of knowing how common these occurrences are. When victims or their survivors have raised legal issues, the cases have often been settled out of court and the documents sealed. It is only when the media attention is brought to bear, as occurred with the extremely high frequency of gallstones in people on low-calorie diets, that victims recognize they are not isolated cases. An article in the *Archives Of Internal Medicine* (August 1989) shows that in eight weeks of dieting on a 500-calorie diet, 25% of dieters developed gallstones.

Side effects of high-protein, liquid-fast diets can include fatigue, depression, sleep abnormalities, cold intolerance, dry skin, dry hair, loss of hair, constipation, delayed emptying of solid food from the stomach, a fall in blood pressure associated with dizziness and even loss of consciousness on standing, and alterations in perceptions of time and space. Generally, there is no mention in the commercial promotions that fatal irregularities in heartbeat could result from prolonged semi-starvation.

Creating a Profitable Addiction

Dr. Stanton Peele, in his book *Diseasing of America*, fully documents as absurd the notion that people who drink too much, eat too much, or spend too much do so because they have an illness. It is his position that "the disease theory of alcoholism and addiction is an elaborate defense mechanism that evades the real issues we face as individuals, families, communities, and as a nation." He believes that providing people with a "lifelong disease" sets them up for relapse and retards personal growth. Dr. Peele believes we are conditioned to fear our environment and conclude we are out of control in it.

So, as a means of escaping our fear and regaining control, we turn to a compulsive behavior and call it a biological disease for which we don't have to be responsible. The treatments for these "diseases" then become our new dependencies, be they medications or lifelong therapy groups. He points out that if excess weight truly were primarily a genetic or biological problem, we would not have a 54% increase in obesity among children age 5 to 11 or a 98% increase in the prevalence of the super obese in this same group since the mid-1960s.

We have more fitness centers and exercise facilities and larger numbers of people using them than ever in the past, but the percentage of people getting heavier keeps increasing. The more treatment programs and doctors working in them that we have, the more weight problems we have. By creating a *disease* diagnosis, we shift the emphasis from social and cul-

tural to individual causes and cures, creating a boom for the weight-loss industry.

Advertisements and doctors convince us we are helpless to deal with our emotions and condition alone, and we buy into a system that not only doesn't solve the problem but makes it worse.

Dr. Peele also brings a great deal more documentation to the idea that compulsively addicted people do much better with their own efforts than by being helped within the medical model or highly structured self-help groups or commercial programs.

Radical treatments, such as those I've outlined here, have been failing for two decades or more, and the libraries are full of independent research indicating that programs and products don't work. Professionals like Dr. Peele and I have written books on why treatments for compulsive behaviors don't work and how they damage possible success. Even former Surgeon General C. Everett Koop pointed out that "quick fix" weight loss does not bring long-term success.

Further Pitfalls of Weight-Loss Diets

We have learned many other things about obesity and weight-loss diets.

- Weight-loss diets are most often diuretic diets and nutritionally unsound, leaving the dieter more vulnerable to illness.
- The quality of medical care in weight-loss programs is most often low.
- Many deaths, illnesses, and emergency operations have been linked to quick weight-loss methods.
- Weight-loss diets are most often boring, bland, complicated, inconvenient, tasteless, strange, or costly, and cannot be continued for a lifetime.
- Dieters seldom stick with a weight-loss diet long enough or consistently enough to lose meaningful amounts of fat, and if they do, they are in danger of harming themselves physically.
- Weight-loss diets often get rid of more lean muscle tissue and water than fat.

- The body has a higher percentage of fat each time lost weight is regained, and the yo-yo syndrome leads to a metabolic condition allowing the body to stay overweight on normal amounts of food.
- Each time a higher weight is achieved, additional fat cells are permanently added.
- After the rapid weight-loss diet is over it leads to a greater volume of food eaten or greater cravings for fattening food.
- Low-calorie diets send the metabolism, thyroid, and sympathetic nervous system down to low gear, depriving nonessential body functions of energy and causing short-term symptoms (e.g., loss of hair) and long-term damage to other organs.

Since this and more is all public knowledge, why do these commercial programs continue to draw large numbers of hopeful clients/patients to still more fat rip-offs?

The effort, time, desire, belief, and hope to do the more difficult things that *will* work have not been emphasized enough to pull the overweight person's attention away from magic bullets.

Showing interest in self-esteem, true healthful eating, overcoming fears and self-doubt, and controlling runaway perfectionism while learning to change taste preferences can seem like too much for one person to take on alone. So why not go one more round trying to beat the odds? Achieving long-term success through a fat rip-off may be expensive and have poor odds for success, but to most people, doing it alone seems even less likely!

Yet there are signs that the numbers of people finding the inner harmony on their own is growing. We are starting to look at those who have made it instead of only those who did not.

Once enough individuals start to believe in and understand themselves and get angry enough to say, "I won't buy it anymore," the whole national problem may turn around rather quickly.

CHAPTER 3

The Weighty Side
Of Perfectionism

Who We Are Might Tip the Scales —
Trim Traits that Last

It is a rare day when Louise appears at work without her beautiful smile, flawless skin, rosy cheeks, and quick, self-abasing sense of humor. She is always interested in the well-being of her close friends and colleagues alike, a hard worker, eager to do more than her share without a complaint and seldom with error. She is modest, sensitive to the feelings of others, and generous to a fault.

It is hard to guess that she is in pain most of the time with a serious back injury, frequent migraine headaches, and a lump in her breast that the doctors monitor closely. Nor would you know that she has a family of four adults at home who count on her to keep everything in their lives together. In return, they provide her with so little intimacy that loneliness is her closest friend. Yet her complaints are few.

Louise's friend, Tomi, is also highly respected at work. Her performance is without fault. She is quick to criticize, but usually not aloud. Her smiles are few and her stoic responses to humor stop most jokes cold. Unlike Louise, she has developed few close friends and does not appear sensitive to the pain of others. Also unlike Louise, she is aggressive and very competitive. At home she kicks the dog and yells at her kids and husband, who can never seem to please her. She controls with an iron hand and complains endlessly about the problems of her life, namely, work, home, spouse, and kids.

Both Louise and Tomi are small in stature and between 40 and 50 pounds overweight. They also have a strong commonality in their personalities. **Both Louise and Tomi, like 85% or more of the clients I have seen for chronic weight problems, are perfectionists.** Louise and Tomi represent different manifestations of the same personality type: the perfectionist.

Like most perfectionists, their focus is outward, watching the world and all in it to see what is expected of them. They are always on guard and ready so as not to fail. Falling short of expectations in any way could mean more than disappointment. For them, the feared result is embarrassment, anger, guilt, shame, rejection, or the ultimate failure: not being loved.

Approval is everything! Most of their motivation and satisfaction comes from outside themselves in the form of approval or perceived rejection. This leads to the belief that their performance is their only worth! Once this idea is established, it is only a question of how to achieve the approval-winning performance.

Each perfectionist may approach this in a somewhat different way, as you can see by looking at Louise and Tomi. Louise is the avoider. She avoids conflict and challenge and pushes her real feelings much deeper than Tomi. She blames herself more, has more guilt feelings, and admits to feelings of inadequacy more easily. She presents herself as more passive and willing to defer and seeks ways to please people as much as possible. Louise feels much more secure and happy when she receives reinforcement that her ways have won acceptance.

Tomi, on the other hand, is aggressive and tries to control rather than defer to others. She focuses on the rules to prove she can't be blamed or officially rejected.

Tomi would fight against admitting feelings of inadequacy, and rather than try to win social approval, she is more apt to use intimidation. She finds it easier to blame others more and rationalize her position. Like Louise, she avoids things she is sure she can't do well. Unlike Louise, she "puts down" those things and the people who do them well. Louise admires and praises those who do what she thinks she would find too difficult.

Overweight perfectionists, like all perfectionists, are prone to have more difficulty with their emotions because they are set up with their own high expectations of themselves and, in Tomi's case, high expectations of others as well. This is especially true of her own children and spouse. Perfectionists are more vulnerable to negative emotions and resistant to change. Tomi looks for things to go wrong and attempts to avoid error by straining to be perfect, which she is sure won't be good enough.

While procrastination is more common with the avoiders like Louise, it tends to be true of aggressive types like Tomi, too. Putting off until the last minute gives less time to prepare. Then, if things don't turn out well, a weak performance can be considered acceptable because of the lack of time for preparation. It won't be considered a failure. If the performance comes out well in spite of minimal preparation, the procrastinator is fantastic. Either way, the perfectionist/procrastinator is safe. There is no risk of failure.

So, if overweight perfectionists are always focused on meeting the perceived expectations of others, and we know that many overweight people tend to be prejudiced against other overweight people, why would the obese person allow him or herself to take the chance of rejection by remaining obese?

Because they have learned that if they work extra hard to please people or to be "right," they are unlikely to be rejected. **If rejection does come, they can blame their obesity.** In the overweight person's mind, the performance — people pleasing — is far more important than any value they may have for the person they are. Because we know the stigma attached to obesity almost assures weak or low self-esteem, which in turn contributes to low self-worth, it is easy to see why a person like Louise is more apt to feel guilty giving herself the same time and attention she always gives to others. Her own physical needs are therefore postponed. We all need approval and praise from others, as well as from ourselves, and if we only get this approval for what we do for others, we may let our own needs slide. In addition, someone like Tomi may believe that if she does achieve a trim body, she'll face new, uncontrollable challenges she could not handle. By holding on to her fat, she avoids facing these challenges.

Perfectionists like Louise and Tomi are more subject to stress and distress, which leads to what Dom DeLuise's cookbook states so profoundly, *Eat This. It Will Make You Feel Better!*

The following quiz is an opportunity to see if you fall into the fat personality group. Give the first answer that comes to mind without considering how it may affect your overall score. If your feeling is both yes and no, go with the one that feels closer. Write your answers on a separate sheet of paper, and ask someone who knows you well to answer the questions with you in mind. Then compare your answers. If the other person has good reasons for an answer different from yours, use it as a chance to reflect on that point about yourself further.

The Fat Personality Quiz

Please answer yes or no to the following questions.

1. Do you routinely set aside your own personal needs to be the best at school or work or to please others?
2. Do people who know you well describe you as a perfectionist?
3. When people around you are upset, bored, or in difficulty, do you feel responsible to fix things for them?

4. Do you frequently contain your feelings to avoid criticism, except at home?
5. Are you quick to criticize yourself or others, or both?
6. Do you usually push to be the best at what you do or avoid doing anything at which you may not excel?
7. When you have a fear that limits the quality of your life, do you seldom *initiate* moving toward the fear to get it resolved?
8. Do you strain, quit, or become very tense when you know you are being compared with others?
9. Do you often feel depressed about your weight?
10. Do you become anxious or bored, especially when you are not productive?
11. Is most change in your life difficult for you?
12. If you lose excess weight, do you wonder if you'll keep it off?
13. Do you want a high degree of structure and time to prepare before you can feel comfortable in new situations?
14. Are you easily hurt, angered, or made to feel guilty?
15. Do you push for control, fear being controlled, fear loss of control, or think you want to be controlled? (If any is true, answer yes.)
16. Have you known yourself to rebel, either openly or otherwise, when you knew it was in your best interest not to?
17. Is anger or physical touching hard for you to deal with?
18. Do you often eat as a response to your emotions?
19. Do you express love, reward, or punish yourself with food?
20. Do you eat more or differently when alone?
21. Do you plan to keep your food taste preferences as they are?

22. Do you benefit (have advantages or security) from being overweight?

23. Do you have less than one enjoyable sexual release each week?

24. Do you believe you'll need help to lose your extra weight and keep it off?

25. Is weight loss more important and urgent to you than changing self-defeating personality traits?

Total the number of "yes" answers. The numbers will indicate the following:

0 - 7	You are likely to stay trim or lose weight easily.
8 - 16	Weight gain may be easy and weight loss very hard to maintain.
17 - 25	Personality trait changes must precede any long-term success in keeping weight in balance with height and build.

The perfectionist personality is not the only aspect of the fat personality; it is simply the most common of the chronically overweight people with whom I have worked over the years. All the questions on the "Fat Personality Quiz" are also aspects that can be found in a variety of other personality groupings, such as the compulsive/addictive types, which also fit with the caretaker/co-dependent, anxiety/depressive types, and certainly, anorexic/bulimic types. None of these classifications, or any other, will fit any one person exactly, or should I say, "perfectly." Each individual is still unique, as are Louise and Tomi, and it is only useful to bring commonalities together under a single label for the sake of clarifying the overall larger problem.

Personality has a great deal to do with why the overweight person procrastinates, drops out, has difficulty staying motivated, or sabotages his or her own efforts. Personality, values, conditioning, attitudes, beliefs, preferences, habits, emotional needs, motivations, choices, and more all run together.

Weight-Loss Myths

My work with overweight people seeking change not only uncovered the problem of perfectionism. It also provided evidence that dispels many commonly held, and sometimes even dangerous, misconceptions about weight loss and individuals who hope to achieve it.

As you read this list, consider how many of these misconceptions you have held or allowed to affect your weight-balance efforts. You'll see that, without exception, debunking these myths supports my belief that any success will come from self-motivation and self-direction, not from outside forces.

- MYTH #1: A family history of obesity cannot be overcome on a long-term basis.
- MYTH #2: Thyroid/metabolic conditions prevent successful weight loss.
- MYTH #3: Poor nutrition and exercise information keep people heavy.
- MYTH #4: Childhood obesity means lifelong weight problems.
- MYTH #5: Victims of child abuse have difficulty losing weight.
- MYTH #6: Giving up smoking or drinking is more difficult than losing weight.
- MYTH #7: The chronically obese must have help to lose weight and keep it off.
- MYTH #8: Once a person has fallen victim to the "yo-yo syndrome" he or she will never be able to lose weight or keep it off.
- MYTH #9: The more weight-loss programs you have participated in, the less chance you have for success.
- MYTH #10: Counting calories is important to long-term success.

Many people I've dealt with have abandoned these myths and gone on to achieve and maintain their desired weights. The next chapter looks at what they've been able to learn.

As long as these myths continue to circulate and remain unchallenged, millions of people will remain stuck within the cycle. Knowing and *believing* the truth can change pessimistic attitudes into optimistic efforts to overcome, individually, what commercial programs promote as a "disease" or condition that cannot be "cured" without outside help.

More than 95% of the people who utilize external motivators or assistance regain their weight plus more within five years (usually much sooner). And that is only if they stay with any program long enough to lose a significant amount of weight to begin with.

But what about those who *do* succeed?

CHAPTER 4

The 5-Plus Club:
A Look at Those Who Keep It Off

Of the thousands of research studies that have been done on weight problems, most take the historical, physiological, sociological, or psychological view that something needs to be cured — as if weight problems are an illness — and that intervention and treatment are the only means of recovery. Few researchers have attempted to examine the possibility that weight problems can be resolved by individuals on their own.

Very few studies have actually examined, or even considered, those people who have lost a good deal of weight and kept it off beyond the time when most people gain it back. Yet the potential to learn something new and valuable is much greater when looking at people who have been successful than by re-examining those millions of efforts over the past 30 years that, generally speaking, have been almost total failures.

Knowing what contributed to the long-term success of others does not mean everyone who follows will also succeed. Nor does it mean that availability of this information will assure that many people will even try to use it. However, it does mean that whoever examines this kind of information has some potentially powerful new choices. It also means that providing this type of information may positively influence previously negative attitudes. Further, it may save some people a great deal of money and help them avoid health risks or make a bad situation worse.

Weight loss is a choice, hard or not so hard, rather than the result of some other factor or combination of factors. It doesn't have a single cause or a single cure. It does not appear to be a disease, nor does it appear to be devoid of sociocultural influences. When those who have succeeded in achieving and maintaining weight loss have been counted, it appears certain they will be far fewer in number than those who have only lost weight.

However, looking closely at the means and methods of those who have succeeded may start a new belief that obesity is more a psychologically intrinsic matter than an illness or genetically predetermined condition, and perhaps more people will make the workable choices sooner.

I conducted an informal study of 30 people to add to what I'd been learning about self-efficacy — the belief in being able to follow free choice in your life — in my 20 years of clinical practice.

All of the people I studied had been overweight, had lost 20 or more pounds, and had kept it off for at least five years. For this reason, I've called them the 5-Plus Club. By looking exclusively at individuals who have been successful in reducing and keeping their weight balanced for five or more years, I was able to verify that most of them did it by themselves and that commercial programs were either of no help or, worse, harmful.

Who Are the 5-Plus Club Members?

This group was made up of seven men and 23 women, ranging in age from 20 to 77. They had all shed between 20 and 170 pounds each.

The number of years members of this group had maintained their weight loss ranged from a minimum of five years to a maximum of 40 years. It should be noted that not all of the subjects sustained 100% of their original weight loss, and not all of them reached their ideal weight.

Nearly half *did* reach their ideal weight. For the other half of the group, though, it continues to be a daily struggle. For this latter half, it is a one-day-at-a-time effort to maintain "control."

Those who are not in a struggle have found a harmony between the emotions they create in their minds and the lifestyle that keeps them trim. For them, it has been a continual process of learning to deal with their emotions and the pressure of their everyday lives.

The onset of weight problems among them was fairly well balanced. A third started during childhood, 1/4 during early adult years (most commonly in the mid to early twenties), and the remainder during the teen years (usually at the onset of puberty). **Sufficient percentages from each age group show that no matter when weight problems begin, including an obese childhood, long-term weight loss is still possible.**

As a whole, the 5-Plus Club is well educated, with most having at least one or more years of college. Members are chiefly outgoing; three-quarters identified themselves as comfortable social mixers. This may indicate a higher level of confidence than in the average overweight person.

Only seven of the 5-Plus Club did not seek help, such as formal programs, in their original attempts to lose weight. Among the other 23 members, outside help was sought one or more times, each time resulting in their regaining what was lost and often more. All but a few of the group were unable to successfully maintain their weight loss until they achieved that loss on their own. This dispels several myths. **One is that the more programs you participate in, the less your chances of success. Another is that yo-yo weight fluctuations prevent permanent loss and maintenance.** Nearly half of the 5-Plus Club members had "yo-yoed" at least two or more times prior to their final, solitary effort. **A third myth this disputes is that chronically obese people**

must have outside help. When members had sought outside help, they were actually unsuccessful.

Bingeing and purging, primarily bingeing, are common among people who use commercial weight-loss programs. With fasting programs, bingeing after the fast is extremely common. A third of the 5-Plus Club had binged prior to their successful last weight-loss effort, and 1/5 had purged. In each case, the purging was usually only done for a short time. Within the group as a whole, *no* bingeing or purging has taken place since their long-term successful effort.

All the members of the 5-Plus Club have substantially reduced their fat intake, and many have become at least partial vegetarians, though only one is a vegan vegetarian (no animal products). **It is reducing fat intake, not counting calories, that determines weight loss.** Only two members of the group found counting calories helpful. Further, calorie counting can become the symbol of control against which many people eventually rebel. It can also create feelings of dependence and lower your reliance on yourself to change.

Similarly, most members who used alcohol or tobacco prior to their successful weight loss have since stopped smoking and drinking altogether. **In each case, they reported that it was easier than changing their eating behavior, which certainly contradicts the myth that losing weight is easier than giving up cigarettes or alcohol.**

Compared with the time when they were overweight, the stability of the home life of 1/3 of 5-Plus Club members has improved. For most of the total group, bringing their weight into balance was just part of balancing the whole of their lives.

A small number of the 5-Plus Club reported being emotionally, physically, sexually, or verbally abused as children. The conventional wisdom is that such people will have much more difficulty in achieving their desired weight and maintaining it. There is some evidence that having been abused as a child does inhibit assertive self-change efforts. **However, the success achieved by these members of the 5-Plus Club demonstrates that once the effort is made, child abuse does not preclude overcoming compulsive behavior over an extended period.**

Eating in response to emotions had been one of the most common characteristics of the 5-Plus Club members at the time they were overweight. Nearly all believed that eating had been a way of dealing with their feelings, and this had become a conditioned response to almost any type of stress. By the time of my informal study, emotional eating was reported by only 1/3 of the group, and everyone had either developed or was in the process of developing new means of dealing with stress.

The amount of stress experienced by this group has also been reduced a great deal. At the time of their peak weights, all but one felt they were experiencing high levels of stress or anxiety. After successful weight loss, 1/3 feel they are under high levels of stress, but how they are handling the stress is much improved.

Perfectionism, quality of home life, stress levels, and emotional eating can all be tied together, so it is not surprising that all but one member saw themselves as perfectionists at the time of their highest weight. At the time of my study, the number of subjects who thought of themselves as perfectionists was reduced to a half, while most of the remainder felt they were significantly less perfectionistic.

Perfectionism is frequently a result of unstable homes. It creates a greater likelihood of high levels of stress and, in turn, contributes to emotional eating. Also, control is a common need of perfectionists, and food is one area of the perfectionist's life that he or she can control. This becomes a good area in which to rebel against one's perfectionism in a passive-aggressive way.

Perfectionism, control, and a need to rebel are also interrelated. Most of the 5-Plus Club members indicated they had been, or continued to be, rebellious. Because they have so often been people pleasers, putting others' needs ahead of their own, they strive to be right by trying to be in control. **Therefore, to submit to something like a structured diet or group plan brings up resentment and rebellious behavior. Overeating is a form of rebellion.**

During their obese years, only 1/3 of my research group felt loved and reported receiving hugs on a regular basis. Today, 2/3 feel they get ample verbal affirmation and touching, and even those who do not, for the most part, feel loved.

Knowledge of nutrition and exercise does play some role in long-term success, but it is not a prerequisite despite what the myth holds. Prior to their successful efforts, nearly 1/2 of the group had little knowledge of nutrition, but by the time they had reached five or more years of balanced weight, only one person in the group felt a lack of basic knowledge about food as it relates to fat. Knowledge of exercise increased even more, with under 1/2 considering themselves aware of proper exercise at the time they began their final weight-loss effort. All of them now feel very knowledgeable about what exercise works for them. This suggests that **when people decide to change their weight and lifestyle on their own, they will seek out the information they need as they need it.**

Depression was common among the group, with most reporting having had feelings of depression related to their weight for the most part. Nearly 1/4 still have recurring, but manageable, bouts of depression. It is interesting to note that most of those still experiencing depression are also still struggling emotionally with their food choices and/or have not retained 100% of their weight loss.

More than 1/2 of the 5-Plus group have been satisfied with their careers, even when they attribute a good deal of their stress to their job. Twenty percent are dissatisfied, and about the same number are neutral, fluctuating between satisfaction and dissatisfaction. Those in the neutral group do not find a great deal of meaning and purpose in their work but are stimulated from time to time. We do know that work can be a major source of stress and, therefore, affect eating and exercise behavior. However, many people who learn how to handle stress with productive outlets and support systems no longer find food a necessary tool for coping.

It is clear from this group that having one or both parents overweight does not mean the child need be overweight. More than 1/2 of the members came from families where either one or both of the parents had a weight problem. In addition, 10 members had reported being diagnosed as having metabolic or thyroid conditions. Yet all had surmounted these supposed roadblocks to successful weight loss. **Even when physical conditions and family history inhibit weight loss, they rarely eliminate the possibility.**

The Motivation for Weight Loss

The motivation for losing weight and maintaining the loss among the 5-Plus Club members is divided into five main categories.

1. APPEARANCE: The number one motivation at the start of the weight-loss effort, and during younger years, was appearance.
2. HEALTH: After five years or more, the primary motivation was health. Just getting older may account for this change.
3. SOCIAL APPROVAL: This held little influence within the 5-Plus Group, indicating the decrease in need to meet social expectations or having met them and indicating an increase in the importance of intrinsic motivation.
4. SELF-ESTEEM: Many did not identify with the need to improve self-esteem, yet after the weight loss and a demonstrated ability to keep it off, members had elevated self-esteem levels more for their self-directed efforts than their weight loss.
5. OTHER: Additional motives included the desire for better sex, more energy, fitness, and the ability to be more active. The motivation still belongs

to the individual even though each person in the group had at least one powerful facilitator. But the facilitator was not responsible for what had happened.

All of the members of the 5-Plus Club have demonstrated intrinsic motivation. Most who reached their ideal weight and maintained it with little or no struggle are primarily intrinsically motivated. The other members of the group are at various levels of developing intrinsic motivation, but they still have, to some degree, an external focus. Some have yet to develop the personal insight, and that might justify a few counseling sessions with an existential counselor (one who facilitates the idea that we all are free to determine much of our life outcomes).

The Importance of an Emotional Support System

One thing at which this group has, as a whole, done exceptionally well is gain emotional support and release. All but one group member used at least one means of emotional release, while most used two or more means of release or support. Ten percent used exercise only (though 3/4 of the group incorporated it as some part of their support system), and one used religion only. Included as one or more of the support mechanisms, in order of popularity, are the following:

1. Exercise
2. Spouse
3. Friends
4. Parents/Siblings
5. Religion
6. Books
7. Meditation
8. Group Therapy
9. Eating Healthfully

Other means used included journal keeping, children, housework, golf, yoga, parties, alcohol, kneading dough, and listening to the radio.

When family members or friends were used for support, it was only as a sounding board or to give encouragement — mostly about stress in a person's life — *not* as a guide or a monitor for weight loss. This is a very important part of the long-term success, but it should not be seen as outside help to control, manage, or even cheerlead. Rather, it should be viewed as a part of a facilitation that comes with a healthful lifestyle, keeping the responsibility, value judgment, and decisions regarding weight apart from the relationship.

It should be noted that exercise gets double, sometimes triple duty. As an emotional adjuster, a calorie burner, and entertainment, exercise plays a vital role that stands out from all the others.

Profiles for Success

What I learned from my informal survey can apply to virtually everyone facing the challenge of controlling their weight.

Members of the 5-Plus Club showed many common characteristics that influenced their ability to master their weight problems. Remember, though, that weight problems have no single cause and probably no single cure. You still must deal with the variety of factors that contribute to your problem and need to be modified in order to resolve it.

The profile that follows is meant only to give the most *common* characteristics of one group of relatively successful people. You will do well to evaluate this information in relation to your own life, viewing none of it as being the perfect answer. **In fact, if there is a single answer, it is that each person has to discover his or her own way.**

Each person in the 5-Plus Club started with different weight and build combinations, different ages and eating habits, different living and working arrangements, different personalities, different genes and conditioning, different parents, different socioeconomic status, etc. They also took different paths to their success. Some people lost the weight in a few weeks. For others it took a few years. Even if the average time is six months, or the most frequent time is several years, it doesn't take into account all of *your* personal variables. The time factor was best measured by looking at the pounds lost per week, which for most was one to three pounds. And this is clearly slower than most overweight people want it to be.

In other words, most of these participants lost their weight in a gradual manner. Learning to be patient and losing weight gradually provided a better chance for long-term success. If you have already developed patience, trying to match the average isn't important. What is important is finding what works for long-term success by looking at all the variables with "gradual" as the guide.

The following profile is *not* set up in a hierarchy of priority. The factors most common to the most successful are noted, as are the successful exceptions. In other words, simply remember that regardless of how common the factors being considered are to the successful 5-Plus Club members, it is still extremely important that you adjust them until they fit *your* use.

The predominant, positive behaviors of the 5-Plus Club members were to:

- FOREGO OUTSIDE ASSISTANCE other than emotional support from friends, spouse, or parents. In the few exceptions where assistance was used, it appeared to have been counterproductive. As long as a quest for external magic goes on, complete, comfortable weight balance seems to be elusive.
- OBTAIN EMOTIONAL RELEASE AND SUPPORT from two or more sources. Exercise and friends were most common, as were lots of hugs and a regular, satisfying sexual release.
- HAVE EMOTIONALLY STABLE HOMES AND SUPPORT GROUPS for themselves that function within a healthful lifestyle of self-development and that are able to lend support in a natural way that

does not control or attempt to assume responsibility for them.

- HAVE GIVEN UP SMOKING, ALCOHOL, OR DRUGS prior to weight reduction, which provided some additional confidence for change as a less stressful first step.
- HAVE ESTABLISHED REGULAR EXERCISE ROUTINES that provided multiple benefits beyond calorie burning and usually were retained more easily than other aspects of lifestyle change. Participating in sports served more as entertainment.
- EAT LOW-FAT OR VEGETARIAN DIETS FOR HEALTH rather than for weight loss. Diets *free* of calorie counting served the highest percentage of the 5-Plus Club.
- BE INVOLVED IN ONGOING EDUCATION, which, whether general or specific to nutrition and exercise, formal or self-taught, served to empower them and give them choices through knowledge.
- HAVE MODIFIED PERFECTIONISTIC CONTROL AND REBELLIOUS TRAITS leading to a more comfortable, less precarious balanced weight. These people were less vulnerable to emotional distress.
- BE PRIMARILY MOTIVATED BY VANITY AND HEALTH to balance weight. Vanity was primary at the start of weight loss, while health served best for endurance. In any case, their motivation was intrinsic, that is, for themselves.
- HAVE A HIGH SATISFACTION LEVEL WITH THEIR CAREER. This seemed to be common to most, together with other major aspects of life (e.g., relationships). Pressure at work was acceptable if satisfaction was high.
- BE SOCIALLY OUTGOING and comfortable with new people and new social situations. However, being comfortable and "doing it" can be two quite different things. A desire or an active willingness to learn to be comfortable is all that is required.

- HAVE REDUCED STRUCTURE AND MORE SPON-
  TANEITY in efforts to change. Finding harmony
  rather than control is the difference between comfortable weight balance and the struggle with
  weight decisions.
- SEEK QUALITY IN LIFE FOR TODAY AND SELF-
  DIRECTED CHANGE FOR TOMORROW. These
  were more common than avoiding change. Common to their success was confronting the fear of
  change that put limitations on life.

Most of these factors have been advocated in commercial and hospital weight-loss settings for at least 10
years or more with the exception of those factors dealing
with outside assistance. **The idea of self-efficacy has
been the missing piece of the puzzle of how weight
losers become long-term successful.** Giving people information only when they have a self-determined need
for the information helps. But setting up structured programs that smack of control and having overweight people pay to have others take the weight off backfire. Even
information regarding motivation, procrastination, and
sabotage only have value in a self-directed effort.

High Self-Esteem Brings Self-Efficacy

I asked members of the 5-Plus Group about such
things as direction in life, change, meaning and purpose,
beliefs, and value priorities to see if these factors influenced their ability to be successful. Approximately half of
the participants felt they were aware of a strong purpose
and meaning in their lives; that is, they had a clear
awareness of their basic beliefs and their top 20 value
priorities.

Change — the Key to Success

Going from chronic weight problems to healthful
lifestyles involves a good deal of risk, which is the point
at which most efforts to change come to a halt. Twenty-
five of this group indicated that they are people who *seek*
personal change, while four tended to avoid change, and
one vacillated.

Desiring and seeking personal change was the single most important factor in the achievement of success within this group. How each person goes about making changes, and how well they continue to do as time goes by, vary a great deal. It is unlikely that any of these people would be in this special 5-Plus Club if they did not have the courage to face the risks of self-directed change.

You can see from the experience of the 5-Plus Club members, from the variety of predominant behaviors they used, and from their different paces of success that no single weight-loss method is best. But you can also see that self-motivation was the key. In the following chapters, we will explore the dynamics of self-motivated weight loss. It is increasingly clear that unwanted weight, and whether or not we can keep it off once we lose it, is a personal choice.

Sometimes, though, we don't make the choice even though we think we want to.

CHAPTER 5

Why Don't I Do What I Think
I Want to Do When I Know
How to Do It?

Louise knows the basics of how to lose weight. Her education in nutrition and exercise, as well as a variety of weight-loss techniques, was certainly more than adequate. She had long been aware of the psychosocial dynamics of the "fat personality." If Louise hadn't changed, it certainly wasn't for a lack of information.

With each new program, method, or technique, Louise planned and organized. She would buy the products and supplies necessary to achieve her goals (e.g., treadmill, books, food). She would go to classes and set up times and places to pull it all together. She would make a consistent effort for a week or two. Her initial enthusiasm would be high and would fade only gradually, usually even after all her efforts had come to an end. In fact, I finally noticed in conversations much later that she would still unnecessarily defend the method and her plan and blame herself for failing.

Louise, as it turns out, did the same things with weight-loss diets, products, or gurus that she did with her parents and sister. When things went wrong, she felt guilty and inadequate. Even in our counseling sessions she would apologize for everything from speaking first or holding a different opinion to taking more than a few minutes to explain her thoughts. If I just looked at her without expression or comment, she would blush, smile her "I'm sorry" smile, become nervous, and stumble over her words. She was acting like a child caught with her hand in the cookie jar, apologizing in a voice that was both short of breath and almost inaudible.

Louise's fear of rejection was plain to almost anyone and more extreme than in most people I see, but what wasn't so clear was the anger that the constricted throat was holding back. The blush, the smile, the apology, and the cute little-girl way of phrasing things all covered up the anger so most people would not notice. **Many other people with fat personalities display their anger, but Louise was the avoider. From early childhood, Louise had been stuffing and eating her anger until it was hard for her to even imagine allowing herself to acknowledge anger, let alone express it fully and openly.**

Millions of people do what Louise did, maybe not in the same manner or degree, but still they do it. They avoid their feelings and deny their anger, only expressing it when it builds to an explosion. When this happens, their anger is usually directed at people they love and are dependent on, usually family members and pets. Playing the role of people pleaser, co-dependent, or caretaker and deferring personal needs for days, weeks, or even years mean building anger, resentment, and frustration. Always putting your needs aside to please others is to feel cheated, unloved, or uncared for. Emotional pressure will build and find some way out, if not in an uncontrolled explosion then certainly in other ways.

The intellect says, "You've learned not to make others angry," so you rationalize not expressing yourself. Since you can't be blamed for what you can't control, you express your anger in a passive-aggressive manner by rebelling and not losing weight. You're innocent. You didn't get mad at *them* directly. You just got back at them by not losing the weight *they* wanted you to.

No, this doesn't make sense, but emotions don't have to make sense. The behavior and emotions keep the mind games going. Even more, they keep the overweight person from dealing with frightening challenges, questions, and problems. Louise's situation illustrates only one of endless ways people can spend a lifetime playing games with their weight. Power, fear, denial, rebellion, control, vengeance, and reward are a few more. They need not have a great deal of logic or reason. But after all, the perfectionists live most of their lives trying to do the "right" thing. Food sometimes seems like the only comfort or sanctuary the perfectionistic person has.

Perfectionists are much more prone to be emotionally stressed, and emotions are a much more powerful motivator than logic. A bright mind can justify (rationalize) staying overweight as being the right thing to do. A perfectionist feels compelled to do what is right or anything to avoid rejection.

Each person has special reasons or circumstances to explain what he or she is doing or not doing. If change is to come, these must be clarified, accepted, and dealt with by their owner. From a base of low self-esteem, it is hard enough just to examine the difficult questions, let alone acknowledge the blocks, identify the means of getting past them, and, in a gradual, self-initiated way, take the action needed to bring about lasting changes.

The Price of Perfectionism

Let's talk about a person other than Louise and look at why, with all the personal differences, one commonality always exists that seems to be the point at which taking progressive, positive action to change stops.

Mr. B puffed with pride. He told me he earned $250,000 a year as an attorney; had a beautiful home; an intelligent, attractive wife; belonged to all the right clubs; bought a new, expensive car every two years; traveled all over the world; and had his two kids in the best colleges. He was also proud that he had graduated near the top of his class at Yale.

Mr. B came into my office defensively, feeling demeaned by being there and attempting to minimize his need for assistance. If 60 extra pounds weren't so hard to conceal, I'm sure he would not have been in my office at all. However, his weight wasn't his only problem. His doctor had also told him that he had hypertension, ulcers, colitis, and, at age 45, he wasn't likely to see 50 if he didn't deal with his weight, drinking, and job stress.

Mr. B told me how his clients, colleagues, and friends loved him and thought he was funny and a master at his profession. Yet his wife was on the verge of filing for divorce, and his kids only talked to him when they needed money.

Yes, Mr. B was a people pleaser, totally focused outwardly, always ready to jump to meet the next expectation. He was highly anxious, depressed, and confused as to why his life was a nightmare. Why was he so unhappy, and why, when he was so successful socially and at work, was his family life so miserable? Unlike Louise, though, he had a litany of blame for other people and situations he couldn't "control."

He was giving me a chance, he warned, but I had better be practical, businesslike, and quick, or he wouldn't be around long. To win his confidence and encourage his efforts, I suggested that he respond to his wife's next daily threat to leave, not by defending himself, but by acknowledging and showing understanding for her complaints and threats to leave. I knew this sudden change would shock and confuse her, and she would back off, at least for a while, which she did.

Mr. B took notes and followed all the practical weight-loss suggestions I made, and, of course, for that period when he was taking those steps, he lost the desired weight. Knowing this small improvement would only be temporary, I gradually started to probe into more sensitive and important matters. As I did so, his defenses would rise accordingly. Eventually, though, he would accept the new ideas and again calm down.

Mr. B acknowledged that he was a perfectionist and a "damn good one." He was proud of it. He had achieved all of his success by being a perfectionist. It was why his reputation at work and the club was so good. He owed "everything" to his perfectionism. Yet it was very hard for him to see the huge price he was paying and had always paid for his perfectionism. It took him a long time to admit his perfectionism was resulting in the following:

- DECREASED PRODUCTIVITY: As many athletes, he did well but always fell short of his capabilities. He was slowed down by attempting precision, being redundant, and missing the big picture.
- IMPAIRED HEALTH: Straining to be the best and fearing he wouldn't be, he was always anxious, not having time to care for himself because it robbed time from his performance for others. The constant strain weakened his immune system and overtaxed his whole body.
- SERIOUS MOOD DISORDERS: High anxiety and depression, loneliness, obsessive-compulsiveness, disordered thinking, and even suicidal thoughts may occur in this kind of self-defeating thinking and behavior.
- POOR SELF-CONTROL: Distress means heightened emotions — the higher the emotions, the less the control. The more unreasonable the expectations and the lower the self-esteem, the more Mr. B saw his difficulties as hopeless.
- TROUBLED RELATIONSHIPS: It is not easy to like someone who is critical, puts himself down, is easily depressed and anxious, and expects others to be as perfect as he thinks he "should" be.
- LOW SELF-ESTEEM: Low self-esteem meant that Mr. B believed his only worth was his performance, and if his performance wasn't perfect, he was a failure. Straining to be perfect, he continu-

ally fell short (at least in his perception). Then he would put himself down, and around it all goes.

- PROCRASTINATION: Because he believed he was likely to fail losing weight (fall short of perfect), he was avoiding doing anything about it. Accepting the price he paid for his perfectionism didn't necessarily mean Mr. B was ready to work on modifying his perfectionistic traits.

Mr. B believed that his perfectionistic behavior and thinking were responsible for his success, and to change could mean he would lose everything, including his wife and kids. It was hard for him to believe that if he were more balanced, with an intrinsic versus an extrinsic focus, lowered his expectations, and was less critical of himself, then he would do even better with work, friends, clients, and money.

He could understand it intellectually but could not internalize it on an emotional level. The only way he ever would be able to internalize it would be if he experienced himself doing things differently. Faced with the fear of changing, Mr. B, like so many others, stopped his efforts and slowly slipped back to his old weight.

Real change means gradually facing your fears on your own terms. We believe about ourselves what we see ourselves do. Repeatedly experiencing new behavior that is self-directed allows us to internalize what we understand intellectually. Then we have changed.

Different people have different fears. For example, some women fear that if they become thinner and more physically attractive they will have men pursuing them. They fear that they might succumb to promiscuity, risking their marriages. In truth, they would be less apt to become promiscuous because they would no longer have to be people pleasers. They would balance their logic and emotions and make better decisions. Self-esteem would be enhanced, and performance would no longer be seen as their only worth. Expectations of others would be decreased, and they would value themselves at a level at least equal to the value they place on achievement.

Excellence versus Perfectionism

If you can modify perfectionistic behavior and thinking, you can achieve excellence, which is a very different and better thing. Perfectionism requires straining, controlling, compulsiveness, and going to extremes that often backfire. You can reach excellence by staying focused on the process, not the outcome, so you will experience patience and balance that bring out the real you. Look at the following list and learn it well enough to make the cognitive shifts that will bring you closer to excellence. Excellence is a high-level wellness. Perfectionism is an unhealthy refusal to accept yourself.

EXCELLENCE		PERFECTIONISM
learning	vs	needing to be right
willing to risk	vs	avoiding fears
empowerment	vs	control
spontaneous	vs	rigidly structured
accepting	vs	critical
sharing	vs	consuming
confidence	vs	doubt
harmony	vs	struggle
journey	vs	destination
involvement	vs	winning
trust	vs	apprehension
evolving	vs	stagnating
loving	vs	struggling to be loveable
high self-esteem	vs	low self-esteem

False Fat Rewards

Many people derive rewards for staying overweight. Thus they fear the loss of these rewards.

- They get more attention from others regarding their helpless position, which can be interpreted as they are loved in spite of their weight.
- Their insecure spouses don't go into jealous rages.
- They are not expected to do as much, especially things they may be fearful of, like the woman

whose mate would like to have her climb moun-
tains with him if she could.
- They fear the loss of power, when size is equated
to power. Size can seem like a means of intimidat-
ing people to control them or get respect.

And on go the reasons people don't do what they
think they want to do when they know how to do it. Each
person has a specific set of circumstances and background to blame. However, when all is examined closely,
it usually comes down to the basics of fear and reward,
which may be the same thing. People are usually afraid
of losing something they have (e.g., a marriage) or of not
getting something they want (e.g., perfection). We will
remain helpless against food as long as we refuse to face
our fears and change the way we perceive ourselves.

Louise, unlike Mr. B, now sees that staying the way
she is, is more painful than facing her fears and changing. By changing, she has a chance of her life improving.
We each have to make these hard decisions, take the
risks, and try again and again until we reach our goals.
Things will only get worse if we avoid facing our fears.

If we try to change outwardly and it goes against our
subconscious beliefs, internal conflict and stress will follow. We would struggle with two motives: 1) to make
logical decisions and act responsibly to apparent needs;
and 2) to avoid aspects of reality that threaten the subconscious beliefs to which we unknowingly cling.

But change we must. Psychotherapy can uncover
what we don't feel safe about letting out. Self-hypnosis
can help us let out deeper beliefs. The chapter discuss-
ing a foundation for wellness will also be helpful.

**Nothing, however, will be as helpful as experienc-
ing yourself behaving in ways for which you can trust
yourself. When you trust, when you feel safe, your
hidden beliefs are released easily.**

CHAPTER 6

Tasteful Seduction

Emotional Eating, Touching, and Sex

Food is sensual, evoking a feeling similar to being touched or hugged; therefore, it is comforting. It is also known that just tasting certain kinds of food — especially sweets, carbohydrates, and fats — triggers a neurochemical reaction in the brain that almost instantly brings feelings of pleasure, comfort, and, at least, a distraction from the concerns of the moment.

Smells hold our strongest memories and are tied to desires and fears, often without our even knowing they are affecting us. For example, when a person wants to lose weight on a conscious level, but has strong memories of food smells that bring back such feelings as family, security, and love, it is hard to turn away from those foods even though they are fattening and damaging to health.

When associations between food smells, love, and security are made, they are more than just memories and desires. They become part of our subconscious beliefs and are capable of shaping and distorting our perceptions. If beliefs of this kind are buried deeply, they become inaccessible and resistant to change. If we do not know what we subconsciously believe, we are likely to act out self-defeating behavior.

From an emotional distance, Louise could clearly see the pattern, the ease with which she had developed the habit of eating in response to her emotions. She was using hugs from the refrigerator in an attempt to fulfill many emotional and physical needs.

Because food can be a tranquilizer and a pleasurable distraction, should this be surprising? In this country, food is available to most of us at any time. Even the poor, whose pleasures might be limited, often find pleasure in food. The food most available to lower income groups is often the most fattening and accounts, in part, for the higher incidence of weight problems among this group.

Eating food is easily justified because it is necessary to life. It isn't usually seen to be as harmful or anti-social as other similar comforters, such as alcohol, drugs, or cigarettes. Being overweight may be looked down on, but eating excessively and inappropriately is encouraged and promoted in every segment of our society.

Louise was not alone in her behavior. Most of the overweight people I have worked with over the years could be regarded as emotional eaters: people who eat to fulfill other than nutritional needs. **The question is not whether emotional eating is a problem. Rather, it is how to change it to pleasurable, healthful eating.**

Understanding how unclarified beliefs and values can be an imperceptible, ongoing source of stress is extremely important to dealing with the big picture as well as to the long-term success for change and weight loss and short-term self-awareness.

Dealing with day-to-day, hour-to-hour urges to eat inappropriately or to avoid exercise requires more self-awareness. It also requires the practice of learned skills to deal with the immediate activities of the mind that we use to drive ourselves.

Louise was very quick to catch on to the process of self-change, but she was very slow to apply her insights. She knew, for example, about what is commonly referred to as *self-talk*. She was aware of *imagery*. And she certainly could understand why it would be useful to monitor her feelings. Louise also knew how to utilize these emotional factors. She eventually decided that this process was important enough to give it a high priority, and each mental activity soon became a part of her consciousness — an ongoing awareness as she needed it. The functional ability to balance and/or utilize her emotions and intellect to her own best advantage helped her in making choices that worked without a struggle.

I want to state clearly that the intent is never to *control* your emotions. Rather it is to utilize them by learning to find a *harmony* between the emotions you create in your mind and your body's physical needs. Control is stressful in itself. Control, like containing, forcing, or straining, fatigues you. **If you attempt to control your diet, you create a struggle in your mind between your will and your emotional desires. The longer the struggle goes on, the more you tire, and the desire to have what you emotionally want quickly exhausts your resistance.**

Harmony is a relaxed, flowing state that brings more usable energy. Harmony moves you in the direction of a natural, healthful response to your body, mind, and spiritual needs, a state of homeostasis or balance, which is the opposite of excess or extreme.

Feelings are, for the most part, generated from our own thoughts, images, past experiences, and behaviors in response to our senses. Emotions are not something that just mysteriously grab us, nor are they only the result of things that happen to us or around us. Moreover, I believe we create emotions by using our ability to speak to ourselves, utilizing mental images, projecting into the future, reflecting on the past, and weighing these factors against our perceived belief of our own ability to deal effectively with the situations and circumstances (imagined or real) that we are facing.

To choose to be fat or thin, it is important to be aware of what we feel when we feel it. As children, we start to learn to suppress our awareness of our feelings because it seems to be socially expedient, and we begin to realize that simply responding to our every stimulus with total abandon isn't especially feasible, useful, or considerate. Nevertheless, disconnecting ourselves from our emotional needs as adults merely to appear bright, quick, and poised is too big of a price to pay.

A Delicate Balance

Knowing what you are feeling (especially a mild feeling) at the time you feel it gives you better choices as to how your feelings will best fit together with your intellectual judgment. When you have a balance between your feelings and intellect, you will find yourself behaving in ways that work to your betterment.

Think of the scales of justice, with your emotions on one scale and your intellect on the other. When intellect becomes greater, emotions lessen. For example, when you are very focused on solving a math problem, not on passing or failing, you have your best chance of figuring it out. But if you wonder or worry about if you'll pass or fail, your emotions interfere, and your chances for failure increase. On another occasion, you may be very turned on to a developing sexual encounter when your partner asks an analytical question. Even if the discussion is brief, figuring out the answer can result in the loss of the sexual feelings you had moments before. Although you may never have a total absence of either emotion or intellect, the more you have of one, the less you will have of the other. The ideal, of course, is a balance.

It is actually simple to gradually redevelop your ability to always be in touch with even your most mild feelings. With practice you will succeed. Ask yourself as many times each day as you can think of it, "What am I feeling?" Listen and your body will tell you. This should only take a split second. If you will, take a moment and practice now! If you tried to analyze your feelings, please try again. You create your feelings in your head, and you experience them in your body.

No doubt you remember your physical sensations when you came close to having a car accident. Your heart may have raced, your stomach turned over, muscles tightened, etc. Your body reacts the same way to less threatening situations, but in a milder way. These mild feelings are the feelings we have learned to ignore.

Think of your body as a barometer. When your feelings are around your ankles, they are very mild. As they build to your thighs, your legs may feel rubbery. By the time they reach your stomach, you have indigestion. At your chest, you have chest pains or a rapid heartbeat. At your mouth, your breath is short or you jumble your words. After your emotions build past your eyes, you are blinded to them, and you are apt to do or say something you will regret later.

Monitoring your emotions gives you some of the awareness you need to keep them in harmony with your intellect. Remember, you always have more than one feeling at any moment. Mixed emotions (a variety of feelings) are not necessarily contrary in making your decisions. For example, excitement and fear may occur together. The more powerful of these feelings may be fear. It holds the most potential because it can lead to the biggest change, as we will discuss later in this book.

Self-Talk

Louise walked to her car after a visit at her doctor. He had been late, his examination of her back had been painful, and she had a headache. If she didn't hurry, she would not have time for supper, or she would be late for her group meeting, or both. The air out in the parking lot was hot, as only September in Arizona can be, and as she approached her car, she saw one of the tires was flat. It was rush hour, she was in the middle of downtown where everything closes by six, and it would be dark in an hour. It was not a safe place to be. Her heart sank into her stomach. In that blink of a moment, she imagined herself unable to locate a towing service, or paying a big fee for one, or trying to fix the tire herself with her dislocated disk, in dress clothes, in 105-degree heat. She could not turn to her husband for help since he was on patrol duty in another part of town. She pictured herself alone in the parking lot after dark, being robbed or raped, and she created a feeling of panic.

The point is, it only took a split second for Louise to become extremely upset. **It wasn't the flat tire that made her upset; it was what she told herself about the tire.** Our minds are faster than any computer in a situation like this. We talk to ourselves and picture in our minds all the horrible consequences that could result from our circumstances.

We talk to ourselves constantly, though we are often not aware of it. We ask questions of ourselves and give answers or debate outcomes. Sometimes we talk to ourselves out loud, and, to me, that only means we can hear ourselves better. What we do with this self-talk can vary a great deal. One thing is certain: self-talk contributes a great deal to creating one's mood from moment to moment. We talk ourselves up or down. We talk ourselves into or out of decisions, and, in my opinion, we even talk ourselves into love. When Louise was in the doctor's office, she was feeling ill, but, not yet knowing about her flat tire, she could still see a way of handling all her concerns of the day. Once she learned of the tire, it all fell apart. Her self-talk raced ahead, and panic, depression, and frustration set in. All of her earlier resolutions about how to deal with her concerns were wiped out.

As it turned out, the husband of one of the nurses was stopping by for his wife and had Louise's spare onto her car in a matter of minutes. Louise laughed about it in her group that evening. She also realized then that she forgot her headache and backache in her anxiety over the situation in the doctor's parking lot. The point is, Louise had a choice about her emotional response to the whole predicament. She could have laughed at the final straw to a bad day and gone back into the office for help, or she could do what she did and create a feeling of panic. Many things could and did influence her choices about creating her feelings, and she also had choices about how she added to or detracted from those external influences.

Pictures of the Mind

In addition to the self-talk that went on in Louise's head, she also created mental pictures that contributed greatly to the resulting feelings. She saw all of the possible negative outcomes of her situation. She saw herself dirty, in pain, paying for a tow truck, getting attacked, being late, hungry, etc. These pictures put a sort of reality to her words that exacerbated her emotions tenfold. **The power of mental pictures is so great that it is hard to estimate the extent of their effect.**

Allow yourself to imagine that you're in your kitchen. You walk to the refrigerator and open it. There, in front of you, is the biggest, most perfect, beautiful lemon you have ever seen. It is flawless. You take it out, and in the warmth of the room moisture condenses on the cool lemon, and little rivulets of water start to pool in your hand. You take the lemon to your counter and cut it into wedges. You pick up the largest wedge and inhale its fragrance. You can see the membrane is bursting with juice. Just by looking at it and smelling it you can already taste it, and you open your mouth wide and bite fully into the lemon wedge. If you have been following along with pictures in your mind, the muscles in your throat contracted, and you puckered or salivated.

This picture story was just to illustrate how powerful mental pictures are in creating emotions. You don't have to imagine lemons, but you can imagine scenarios, behaviors, and attitudes that will benefit you. Feelings are created by mental pictures about almost everything we worry about or look forward to. You can use your mental pictures for or against yourself. If you are going to utilize your mental pictures to your advantage, again, it will be as a result of your practice and learned skill.

Start by picturing some of your favorite places where you feel safe and comfortable. These can be places you have experienced or ones you've created, just so you find pleasure in them and want to return. Practice frequently by exploring the details of the scenery, focusing on the clarity of the picture, and employing your senses. For example, see yourself at the beach. The temperature is ideal, and you're seated in the sand. You feel the warmth of the sun on your body and the cool breeze on your skin, and you smell the sea water. You feel the soft sand underneath you. Pick up a handful of warm sand and notice the grains separate and flow through your fingers. Only a few people are there, and the scene is tranquilizing. You notice the sharp, bright colors of the swimsuits, the sizes of the bodies, the ages of the people, the shells and seaweed on the shore, and the sound of the waves as they break against some large rocks. The sound of the children at play in the surf suggests how good the water would feel. This becomes a vivid picture full of details and brings your senses into play.

The more you practice mental imagery, the more you can use your fantasies and dreams to your advantage. By monitoring your emotions, self-talk, and mental pictures, you will find you are better able to find a calm harmony within yourself and a growing confidence about your ability to deal with the situations of your life.

Beliefs, values, decisions, monitoring emotions, self-talk, and *mental pictures* are basic aspects of self-directed change in the long term and of day-to-day emotions and behavior in the short term. Once you have the ability to utilize these factors, other parts of your life will come together so your self-esteem and other common traits of the fat personality will be modified. It will never mean the removal of all stress from your life, but the incidents of distress that may lead you to the refrigerator will be fewer, and you will handle them in a very different, self-enhancing manner. Self-esteem needs are met here (e.g., knowing what you believe, value, and feel; making decisions that fit; being responsible for your feelings and thus your behavior). It is the positive time, attention, and energy you give to yourself that raise your self-worth, trust, and self-efficacy, just as you must meet your basic human need for sex and touching.

Touching Power

Touching is now known to be a necessary element in human growth and development as well as to promote a healthy immune system. Volumes have been written on the statistical, experimental, and clinical research that has been done on the subject of touching. However, it is still unusual to find a question about touching on a medical history or stress-assessment questionnaire, which may testify as to how uncomfortable our society is with the subject. It's a sad and common reality that the only time some people are touched is by paying for it, such as by the chiropractor, the hair dresser, or a professional massage person. Even many health practitioners, such as doctors, nurses, or counselors (who know the healing power of touch) are afraid to touch or hug their clients or patients because they may be misunderstood and sued for making improper advances.

After the honeymoon period of marriage wears off, husband and wife frequently only touch during sex or in parting or arriving home. Children, all too often, are deprived of parental touch after reaching adolescence.

Touching is a part of communication. It is a means of being reassured that we are cared for and loved. It can provide us with a sense of security and well-being that assures us in ways words can't always do. It is easy to understand how, in a critical, competitive society such as ours, true intimacy is hard to find. It may seem safer or easier to get our hugs from the refrigerator. Because we reserve touching for special occasions, we lose awareness of its larger values and forget its importance and connections to the needs in our day-to-day lives.

The longer we avoid that which we need or fear, the greater the chance we will become paranoid about it or pay a price for it in illness or pain. People who like themselves for who they are and not just for their performance will be comfortable with touching and intimacy and automatically accept and initiate it as a natural, valued experience.

Real hugs can alleviate much of the need for hugs from the refrigerator very effectively.

Louise was not getting enough touching at home, and this lack not only contributed to her weight problem but also to becoming involved in extramarital affairs, separation from her husband, and possible divorce.

Food is sensual, as is sexual activity, and both eating and engaging in sex can lead to a temporary calming. Therefore, it is easy to see how people can substitute one for the other and never notice the substitution is being made. The healthy human body prepares itself many times each day for a sexual encounter. Even though age has a bearing on frequency, the biological phenomenon can last throughout our lives, barring illness, excessive stress, or fatigue. If we seldom respond to our libidinous drive, a sexual tension builds that needs some outlet.

We have commonly cut ourselves off from our milder feelings as a result of our social fears, stigmas, and competitive drives for security and approval. So recognizing or attending to our sexual needs tends to take a low priority on our motivation and value scale. It can be easy to find yourself haunting the refrigerator for snack food a hundred times over and never make the connection between your sexual needs and the unexplained, unquenchable appetite. Rosalyn Meadow and Hillie Weiss elaborate on this subject in their book, *Conflicts About Eating and Sexuality.*

The only times I've seen people recognize some relationship between sex and eating is when the exchange goes to an extreme, where intercourse has stopped for a long period of time, and eating rituals have become more elaborate and exotic, evolving into a clear sexual medium between partners. This is well depicted in the movie, *The Loved Ones,* when the character Joy Boy, played by Rod Stieger, has a vicarious, incestuous relationship with his morbidly obese mother.

But emotions, and how we learn to deal with or sublimate them, are not the only way we can change.

CHAPTER 7

Beliefs, Values, Decisions —
A Foundation for Wellness

The Basis for Change

Like almost all the people I've seen over the years, Louise was lost when I asked the question, "What is your philosophy of life?" No matter what the person's station in life, age, IQ, profession, or income level, I have yet to get more than a flip or singular answer to my question. It isn't that people don't have a set of beliefs; it is more that they have never analyzed the basis and concepts they use for expressing their fundamental beliefs. They may have an overall vision or an attitude toward life and its purpose, but they don't consciously know what it is.

As a college student, I remember being asked on employment forms about my philosophy of life. At that time, it all seemed irrelevant, and I would write whatever came into my mind just to get it out of the way. Now, after helping hundreds of people to change their lives for the better, I realize one's philosophy of life is basic to intrinsic change.

To me it is like wanting to go on a trip to a specific destination. But not knowing where I am, it is then awfully hard to determine the direction to travel. If I don't know who I am, how can I know what to change to become what I want to be? Most clients are able to give me a chronology of their life, but they aren't clear about who they are as a person. This lack of self-knowledge suggests a lack of value they have for themselves, and this is commonly a major part of the problem.

Like Louise, most of us have been so busy trying to live up to what we imagine others expect of us that we have not had time to be concerned with who we are. It has simply been to get on with the next task to reach the next goal. To do otherwise seems frivolous and produces guilt. In the case of Louise, with her sense of low self-worth, taking time to nurture her own well-being would take away from her external focus (as caretaker/people pleaser) and threaten her security. So she just keeps plowing ahead, not knowing why or if her actions fit with her beliefs.

Part of my conviction is that everything we do, think, and feel comes out of our beliefs directly or indirectly. Our beliefs influence every aspect of our lives every minute of every day we are alive. Beliefs are the basis for our motivation to do, or not to do, anything. If part of what I believe is that my performance is my only true value or worth in life, then I believe that if I can't do many things — or even one thing — I'm apt to be rejected (not loved). Therefore, it would be easy for me to become a perfectionist and not know why. However, I don't have just one belief. I have many, a set, or system of beliefs about almost everything I've encountered. Even if my reaction is "I don't understand," then that is my belief. We don't escape our beliefs, but we may not be aware of them.

Here is one more illustration to make my point. Think of yourself as a loan manager at a bank. With your signature alone, you are authorized to lend $50,000 of the bank's money. One of your many beliefs may be that humans are basically evil or basically good, or your belief may be that humans simply have the potential to be good or evil. It doesn't take much thinking to realize that no matter what you believe in this instance, it will clearly affect the way you do or don't give out loans. Even though in this position, with the approach of each new loan applicant, you aren't consciously thinking that people are good or evil, your decision as loan manager will be influenced by this basic belief. Now project from this one belief to all your beliefs, and you begin to see how powerful your beliefs are in determining your every thought, behavior, and feeling.

Also out of beliefs come the meaning and purpose in life. The better we understand our meaning and purpose, the better we can handle the difficulties of life. Once you are able to understand why you are struggling with something, you will be able to endure more and feel better about doing it. A good example is prisoners of war or hostages. In the past, some have been known to give up under their hardships because they didn't know why it was worth continuing to struggle. It is possible for a person under these conditions to simply curl up in a corner, never move again, and die. Others, like Victor Frankl, as described in his book *Man's Search for Meaning*, discovered a meaning and purpose under such horrible conditions, and in their own way made it through, often sustaining greater hardships than those who died. Some, like Dr. Deepak Chopra, hold that beliefs and emotions influence every cell in our bodies, creating illness and health.

Approaching Real Self-Awareness

It is also my conviction that when our beliefs are not clear to us, it is like a void or empty space inside us. When our beliefs are not clear to us, they are unknown, and unknowns about ourselves produce a low-level, ongoing anxiety. Over time the anxiety becomes almost imperceptible to us. Our state of mild anxiety becomes so familiar that it seems normal or usual. To suddenly feel fully calm, then, might seem strange or even frightening. Ongoing low-level anxiety, unlike the anxiety we experience when we almost have a car accident, wears us down. Our immune system weakens, making us more subject to illnesses, and we are more vulnerable to experiencing distress from vicissitudes that may befall us day to day. We react to new problems more often, more quickly, more strongly, and our reactions last longer when we have continuous low-level anxiety. Of course, more emotion means more need for comforting from that sensual nemesis — food. More *Hugs from the Refrigerator*.

Having your philosophy of life clear in your mind will go a long way toward reducing anxiety by building confidence and filling up the internal void. It will also get you started clarifying your value priorities since they are built on your beliefs.

Use the following philosophy-of-life organizer; plan to take your time, be patient, and follow the steps to get clearer about the base your life is built upon.

Your Philosophy-of-Life Organizer

Figuring out a philosophy of life requires time, reading, observing, experiencing, reflection, frequent discussion, writing, and rewriting until you are clear with yourself. Some people make the mistake of assuming that this task can be done off the top of their heads in five minutes. If that's the time they give it, that's exactly how deep, meaningful, lasting, and valuable it will be to them.

In reality, there is no set way to uncover your personal philosophy, and the project will never be completely finished; however, by establishing a base point, each person can be on top of his or her beliefs, values, and gradual changes as life is experienced. We can be much more sure of who we are, which is invaluable in reaching our goals.

Consider the following guide for helping illuminate your beliefs. Each premise comes from my belief that we can change our lives and speaks of an important factor in a person's philosophy of life. Evaluate each, then consider a personal belief you hold about it. On a separate sheet of paper, change and add material until you've developed a philosophy with which you are comfortable. But remember, you are always in a state of becoming. What you are becoming has a great deal to do with your beliefs. You are free to choose that for which you can like yourself. Consider these few examples, which are no more right or wrong than your own ideas. You can use these to prime your interest.

- We have free choice (i.e., to be fat or thin). What do I choose to be as a person?
- Purpose and meaning are essential to inner peace, happiness, and endurance. What gives purpose and meaning to my life?
- We each determine our own truth. What do I hold to be true about life?
- Movement (change) is life (living, growing, dying). In what direction do I want to go today and tomorrow?
- Love is the most powerful force. How would I describe my ability to love?
- Questions, challenges, and problems are essential to a positive self-image. What questions, challenges, and problems have priority for me?
- Humans have potential to be good or evil and are free to determine what is good or evil. By what standards do I measure good or evil?
- All things are connected — all things can lead to something better. What aids my ability to function in harmony with other things and grow from discord?
- All people are unique or special and yet the same. What is my special uniqueness?
- Reality and illusion can be the same. What might my imagination lead me to?
- Self-identity comes from observations, comparisons, decisions, and responses to experiences. How does my self-identity develop?
- Balance or centeredness brings out human potentials. What brings me a sense of stability?
- Individuals often misinterpret or ignore their own motivations. What are my value priorities?

Question your own beliefs as you go and make adjustments on each new draft until you run out of new
questions and thoughts.

Then write your final draft and reread it until you
can verbalize it without the aid of your draft. Gradually,
you will come to notice changes in your beliefs as they
are happening. If you really do clarify your own beliefs in
this manner, it will significantly change your life even if
you don't incorporate any of the other self-enhancement
suggestions offered in this book. You will be calmer,
more thoughtful, more decisive, more understanding,
more fulfilled, more honest, more authentic, and more
successful.

Your Value Priorities

Knowing your value priorities is the second part of
self-awareness necessary to the process of self-directed
change and eventually good health through balanced
weight. This section will guide you to developing your
own list of values as you see their priorities. Getting your
values clear and in a usable order will take time, effort,
and a good deal of reevaluation. If your interest and
belief in these priorities are not there, if identifying, cate-
gorizing, and prioritizing are not a *high* priority with you,
return to it another time. Just going through the motions to say you have completed the task would be of
little value to your change process.

Think in terms of writing three to six drafts before
you are comfortable with knowing what is important to
you. Ideally, between drafts, there would be a great deal
of thought and discussion with those who know you
well, and observation and dissection of all aspects of
your life. **You should also compare the manner in
which you actually use your time to what you believe
is most important to you.** Reflecting with people who
know about what you have done helps you to value the
changes you've made. It also helps to follow this reflection on the past with projection into the rest of your life
in an effort to imagine changing needs and activities
before finalizing your values.

No matter how "perfect" your priority list, time and experiences will require you to question your values, and modification will be likely. However, once your values are a part of your consciousness, you will notice your changes as you make them. The closer you come to living by your own value priorities, the more you will trust yourself and the less you will have doubts about what you can or can't do. For example, once you see health as a top priority, you will be better able to deal with the urge to eat something you know works against you, that doesn't fit in your value system.

Remember, your beliefs are the base upon which your values are built. Like beliefs, if your value hierarchy is unclear to you, you may create an almost imperceptible anxiety within yourself. By continually choosing lesser values over your more important values, you may not even notice a problem until you are paying a price you'd rather not pay. If you commonly choose value number 20 over value number two, and you aren't aware of it, you will find it hard to relax or to like or trust yourself.

Being aware of ourselves includes being aware of what we believe life is about and the order of importance that ideas, people, property, experiences, etc., have to us. Start with the most important things (other than life itself) and work down to at least value number 20. In other words, if you had to give up everything in your life except one thing, what would that be? Your children, parents, spouse, your career, your health, your religion, etc., etc.? Whatever it is, that is your first value priority. Keep going until you have your top 20. You'll notice before you finish that your priorities all overlap. And somewhere among them, probably near the top, you will probably find values for good health and nutrition.

If you are wise, you will take your time, rethink your choices, and go over them again and again. You have already changed them many times in your life. Now you want to have them clear day-to-day, knowing when and why they change. It will help you to be emotionally stronger and better able to establish direction in your life — even to find meaning and purpose in what you are doing with your life. Most of all, this knowledge will enable you to make better decisions — decisions you make every day, all day, from the time you become conscious each morning until you fall asleep each night.

Not only are we constantly deciding about something, but each decision also affects our self-image. **When our decisions are in keeping with our values, we like ourselves better, we trust ourselves more, and we fear our decisions less.** We don't have to be perfect, and, therefore, we come much closer to our potential to be happy, loving, insightful, creative, kind, giving, bright, and physically healthy — and, yes, maybe even to be more successful. With your beliefs and value priorities clear in your mind, monitoring your decisions that lead to your improved self-image will go more smoothly.

Begin making your list of value priorities on a sheet of paper. Start with what is most important to you and work your way down to 20 items. Also give careful consideration to whether a value you list is truly important to you or whether it is something you have been trained to value. For example, a young mother would probably pick her child as her first priority. But if she considers this she'll realize that her own mental and physical health will determine how much she can give her child. It may be against her training to put her own health first, but it is the way she will be able to give the most to her child.

Remember that your list will change as you give it more consideration and as you reflect more on your day-to-day experiences. But after several versions you will come up with a list that is a true representation of your value priorities.

Once you've done this, estimate the amount of time and effort you devote to each value. Then compare this with where each value falls in your priority list. If you're devoting a disproportionate amount of time or effort to a

value that is low on your list, you should consider finding ways to redirect yourself to better match your priorities. For example, if you frequently drive your children to
dance class and baseball practice, how much time do
you allow for your own exercise? *The Book of Questions*
by Gregory Stock can be useful and fun in groups to help
clarify your values.

Going to the "Plate"

Louise was keenly aware of which foods were most
healthful and least fattening, but she would routinely
choose fattening food as she went through her choices at
restaurants, the grocery store, and while holding open
the door of her refrigerator. When you imagine how many
times she made these choices over the years, even after
she became aware of the truth about her choices and
knew that one of her highest value priorities "should" be
her health, you can imagine how her view of herself was
being chipped away every time she ate fattening, unhealthy food. The message to herself was, "Louise, you
can't trust yourself, and your own life isn't as important
as all the people you care for." By acting contrary to her
own values, she came to believe she couldn't put faith in
her ability to choose based on them.

The occasions on which she would make healthful
choices, of course, would somewhat balance out the self-
defeating choices, so the whole process became like a
batting average. The more times she went to the "plate,"
the harder it was to change her batting average. When
Louise's choices were predominantly self-defeating
(against her health/weight values), her self-image
dropped more than it raised. Now, if you think about all
the other choices (decisions) in her life that are aligned
or opposed to her own beliefs or value priorities, you can
see how her total self-image moves up and down.

What we witness ourselves doing as a result of our
decisions becomes what we believe to be true about who
we are. Again, it took time for Louise to change a view
she held about herself; it was gradual and involved most
aspects of her life. She had to be more sensitive and

self-aware so she could realize new self-enhancing choices. Most of all, to turn around her self-image, she had to be patiently brave, calling upon her courage, in spite of her own poor image of herself, to face the hard decisions, take the risk of failure, and do it over and over until the changes created a new and improved view of herself that she believed.

Beliefs, values, and decisions are the basis for self-change and interact with all the things you might do to achieve the trim body you seek. A number of the other basic things on which you will test your beliefs, values, and decisions will be covered in the chapter on stress. Remember, you don't have to do it all at once. Please do not try. All parts of the whole (you) are important, and the more you bring them together, the faster your desires will be attained.

CHAPTER 8

De-Stressing Distress

Stress, the resulting socioemotional behaviors, and the lack of coping or adjustment skills are primary aspects of my wellness theory of weight gain and loss. They have been key to my philosophy for a long time. In fact, many of the key elements were presented in my earlier book, *Change Your Mind/Change Your Weight* (Health Plus Publishers, 1985).

Emotional eating patterns vary among individuals. Some individuals will be unable to eat if experiencing any amount of stress; others eat more when their stress levels are escalated. This was the case with Louise. Depression, loneliness, sorrow, joy, or excitement at a high or low intensity usually meant she would eat more.

Fear and anxiety are by far the emotions most commonly responsible for sending people to the refrigerator for a hug. Whenever a person perceives a threat to his or her security, desires, needs, or wants, he or she is apt to realize some type of physical and/or emotional response that could be classified as stress. Our neurochemical systems (when functioning well) react to all changes in our environment with some degree of stress, but it is when we consciously perceive a change or possible change, and we question or doubt our ability to cope, that our stress symptoms appear and our ability to function at our best is impaired.

Even positive emotions such as excitement, happiness, or joy can be stressful. Your body does not distinguish between the types of emotions you are experiencing, only the degree of intensity and duration. Physical injury or illness produces stress, as does excessive fatigue, obesity, or the trauma of exerting vast reserves of energy. In all these instances, your body and mind prepare to defend themselves, balance themselves, or flee.

What is stress, then? It is your physical and mental reaction to your real or imagined environmental changes and the perceived threat to your survival or equilibrium. Your senses bring you messages; your brain measures them; your mind determines if you can handle them; your body reacts. There are three forms of stress: *usable stress* (for example, superior recall of rehearsed lines while performing on stage), *manageable stress* (such as controlled but unimaginative job interview responses) and **distress** (for example, deliberate binges as a result of a perceived inability to cope). It is the last, distress, that you will learn to manage and control.

Recognizing Symptoms of Stress and Distress

Remember, some symptoms are too slight to be noticed. Some symptoms we have either disconnected ourselves from or have suppressed because we mistakenly think they interfere with the way we want to be perceived by others. Some symptoms are noticed more by others than by us. Some symptoms demand that we take notice, and these are the ones with which we are most familiar. Many times while being measured for stress levels, biofeedback clients have told me they felt very relaxed (and they believed it) when the feedback was clearly fairly high on the stress scale. Many of us have become very skilled at blocking our own responses.

Symptoms can be almost as many as there are people, circumstances, and things to which to react. The following are typical symptoms of stress and distress:

- Illness — anything from allergies to cancer.
- Disordered thinking.
- Hypertension.

- Chest pain.
- Excessive drinking.
- Difficulty in sleeping or relaxing.
- Speech impairments.
- Poor concentration.
- Nervous tics.
- Hyperactive behavior or speech.
- Lack of joy found in entertainment.
- Loss of sense of humor.
- Low sexual interest or sexual dysfunction.
- Vision problems.
- Muscle or structural problems.
- Rapid heartbeat, pulse, or breathing.
- Paralysis.
- Loss of energy.
- Short temper.
- Loss of interest in old pleasures.
- Frequent withdrawal.

Sources of Stress

Causes of stress are as many as the many changes that occur in our lives. Any change perceived by our senses or imagined by our mind can be stressful. Some stress is generalized, some is very specific. Some stress is learned and becomes a conditioned response; some comes through trauma or shock. Pollution, the economy, traffic congestion, war, crime, jobs, unemployment or the threat of it, romance or the lack of it, body image, injury, drinking, smoking, poor diet, children, or parents can be the start of an endless list of what are called *stressors*. For many people with weight problems, one of the biggest stressors is perfectionism. The pressure to be perfect creates a vicious distress cycle. The more stressed we are, the more dissatisfied we are with ourselves, and the more likely we are to engage in overeating.

What you believe about your environment and your ability to cope have everything to do with how you create usable stress, manageable stress, or distress.

Distress Prevention and Stress Management

Prevention and management of stress and distress are important for people who seek wellness as much or more than weight loss. The quality of your life, and of those in your life, is greatly enhanced by the practice of the following basic wellness habits. Once a stress storm is in progress (and it can be manifested as eating) learning or utilizing these practices is of much less value. It's rather like installing the smoke detector during the fire.

Think of these practices as adding to your life in terms of quality and achievements. The important aspects of stress management are:

- SELF-AWARENESS: Become aware of the connection between what is happening in your mind and body in relation to your environment. This is a natural ability that you can relearn simply by practicing listening to yourself and becoming aware of yourself until it becomes a habit that is done without conscious effort. Candid discussion and feedback from others who know you are also helpful.

- EXERCISE: Establish a frequent (four or more times a week), varied routine that is safe, progressively more vigorous, and balanced (including stretching, contracting, and aerobic exercise), with satisfactory recovery time in between.

- REST: Take time for sufficient sleep (a full eight hours, which is more than most adults think they need). Dreamwork, waking fantasy, and calming practices such as meditation can also be useful.

- NUTRITION: Know what food is doing to you. If you eat a food that is not healthful, not only will you add physical stress but you will cause emotional distress as you realize you have acted against your values. By changing to a more healthful eating routine, you can reduce your stress on two levels.

- SUPPORT SYSTEM: Develop emotional, social, career, and physical support from organizations, personal beliefs, secure places, and friends and loved ones who appreciate you, nurture your development, and are working on their own healthful lifestyles.

- CALMING ACTIVITIES: Enjoy pursuits that add to your well-being and strengthen your resolve to change. We all must find our own calming activities. Putting my thoughts on paper is one of mine; walking with a special person or alone is another. For some people it's fishing, art, music, etc.
- ENVIRONMENT: Make sure your surroundings include clean air, full-spectrum light, enough space, comfortable noise levels, pleasing colors, safe radiation and radon levels, safe building materials and furnishings, etc.

Making these factors part of your lifestyle will keep a good deal of stress from becoming distress and will enable you to capitalize on useful stress. It isn't helpful to strain to be perfect in all these areas, but simply to give them a priority when the choice is yours.

De-Stressing Stress

The movement from stress to distress may be slowed, stopped, or reversed simply by using the following self-analysis. If you have incorporated the prevention methods indicated above into your lifestyle, the following steps will be a quick, practical exercise for you.

- ACKNOWLEDGE YOUR FEELINGS. When you acknowledge your feelings, you are in touch with them and admit *you* have developed them. Being out of touch with your feelings is not a lack of intelligence or any other flaw in you; rather, it is learned behavior that you can change through awareness.
- IDENTIFY YOUR EMOTIONS. Do they include anger, fear, hurt, frustration, joy, peace, love, sexiness, hate, calm, excitement, etc.? The more accurate you are in identifying your emotions, the more effective you can be in dealing with them.

Remember, you're likely to be experiencing more than one emotion at any moment.

- DETERMINE THE LEVEL OF THE FEELINGS YOU ARE EXPERIENCING. Which feelings are slight? Which are strong? Are you only ill at ease, or are you about to lose what you think of as "control"?
- ASSESS WHAT YOU ARE DOING WITH THESE FEELINGS. Are you straining to make them go away? Is your self-talk building up the feelings or toning them down? Are you pushing them into your subconscious? Are you examining them closely and dissipating them? You're the boss!
- DETERMINE THE SOURCE YOU ARE USING TO CREATE YOUR STRESS. Are you giving a conditioned response? Are you creating stress about something you predicted would happen? Is the source something new and confusing that you fear you may not be able to deal with? Is it something from inside or outside yourself (for example, physical pain you can't explain versus someone trying to sabotage you at work)? Is your stress about survival (food, air, health)? Is it the unknown? It may take some intellectual detective work to determine the source you are using to create your stress, but the deductive process itself will reduce stress. Finding the cause can help you to understand why you've chosen to create the stress and will give you better options for dealing with it effectively.
- EXPRESS YOUR FEELINGS POSITIVELY. Finding a positive expression for your feelings is the last step in reducing stress. All of these steps are part of self-awareness, and as your level of reasoning increases, your emotional stimulation goes down.

If, however, you have a residual amount of emotion to dissipate, express your feelings in ways that won't hurt you or others (nor cause others to defend themselves). Raise your voice or really yell. As long as you are not blaming others or putting them down, most people can deal with a little noise, and you feel better. Expend physical energy. Run, jump, or hit *soft* things that you can't hurt and that can't hurt you.

Look in the mirror and "sincerely" strain to look and feel as upset as you can. It becomes a paradox; the harder you try to look and feel upset, the harder it is to stay upset. Visualize in your mind or write in a letter you won't send what would be self-defeating if you did it openly.

Principles of De-Stressing

The techniques you can use to de-stress yourself are almost as unlimited as those stressors you've acquired to stress yourself. If any stress-reduction technique is to have a good chance of being useful to you, the practice of it will be initiated by you, without predetermined judgments, but rather with an open mind to possible outcomes. It will be practiced with great regularity, and it will be most helpful to you if it is created or modified by you to meet your special circumstances. The elements listed below are often useful.

- LET DOWN YOUR DEFENSES. Allow your mind to be quiet. Relax your muscles. Reduce sensory stimuli — sight, smell, taste, sound, hearing.
- HAVE A FOCUS AND KEEP IT SIMPLE. Your focus can be external or internal. It can be imagined or real. Use one of your senses to focus on a movement, an object, a sound, a color, a smell, or a taste that is healthful and that you're learning to like. Or focus on something such as your breathing. Try not to be distracted or to think of anything other than the selected focus.
- CHOOSE A SAFE PLACE. It is important, especially at the start, to practice de-stressing activities where you feel sure you'll encounter no interruptions, danger, or distractions. As you progress, you will be able to tolerate more stimuli. Build your confidence first.

- TRY TO HAVE AN EMPTY STOMACH AND A
  RESTED BODY. An active stomach makes it hard
  for your mind to relax. Being tired and ready for
  sleep means you probably will fall asleep rather
  than practice stress relief. You may not be aware
  of your stress while you're sleeping, but you will
  have done nothing to eliminate it. It will be there
  when you awake.
- ALLOW YOURSELF TO RELAX. Straining to relax
  creates a paradox. Push, force, and strain to relax, and you become more tense. Strain to stay
  awake, and you fall asleep. Just "letting go" of
  your mental struggle or conflict is the key to
  achieving relaxation.
- BE AWARE THAT THE MAGIC THAT WILL ALLOW
  YOU TO RELAX IS INSIDE. You hold the key to
  relaxing. The key is to practice *before* the emotional storm. External, quick fixes are temporary,
  habit forming, dangerous, lower your opinion of
  yourself, and end up creating more stress. The
  sooner you quit looking for the magic outside, the
  sooner you will find it inside.
- FIND YOUR HARMONY BUTTON. The relaxation
  technique most apt to work for you is the one that
  appeals to you most — the one you believe in. You
  will be able to shorten the process so that a single
  "cue," such as a certain word, sound, movement,
  image, or color, is all you need to slip into a relaxed, harmonious state.

When you are learning a relaxation technique, remember, it is more than the *technique* you are trying to
learn, and it is even more than the ability to relax you
are after. **You are trying to change your self-image by
demonstrating your willingness to consistently give
the time and energy you need to follow through on
your commitment to yourself.** This means you will do
this even when you don't feel like practicing and when
requests from people you care about could easily take
you away from it. If you consistently, but not rigidly,

nurture your own skill in this manner over a meaningful period of time, you will not only master the task, but you will also increase your self-esteem, self-worth, self-confidence, and self-trust. This all translates into less doubt about whether you will or won't eat and exercise in a healthful manner.

The rate at which you develop mastery of any method or technique depends on your personal history and the circumstances in which you work, play, and live. Some people are afraid to relax. To them, relaxing feels like loss of control. Others get too excited about the possibility of relaxing. Some doubt themselves and fear failure so much (a manifestation of perfectionism) that they give up quickly. And some pick it up quickly simply by permitting it to happen, without self-doubt.

Relaxation Facilitators

The following techniques are a small representation of the hundreds that are known to facilitate relaxation. However, most anyone can probably find at least one acceptable technique on the list. Again, as with menus and recipes, those that you modify or create are the ones that you are most apt to use, value, and practice the longest. Most of these methods are simple and require little or no equipment or investment other than your own effort. The basics of a few suggested techniques may best be learned with the help of a professional or someone you know who is practicing them.

WATER: The movement, sound, and temperature of water seem to have a relaxing effect on most of us. Watching water, listening to waves or rain, riding on a ferryboat, or slipping into a warm bubble bath or hot tub is almost certain to take the stress away from most of us.

MOVEMENT: This includes dancing, running, walking, yoga, stretching, aikido, Tai Chi, Feldenkrais, etc. Movement will release stored energy, allowing for relaxation. Aerobic movement generates endorphins, helping relieve anxiety and depression. Movement also helps to change your focus and thought process. It was here that Louise found her solution to stress, as you will see.

MINDLESS ACTIVITIES: These can also provide focus and movement to help you relax. Whittling, rubbing a worry stone, and doodling are examples requiring little or no thought, talent, or training. Counting down is especially good for relaxing or going to sleep. Count down from 1000, visualizing each number. Also, with each number, inhale slowly and fill your lungs, then breathe out in the same manner during each count. With both your body and your mind working together and occupied, stressful thoughts are unavailable, and you relax.

ART: Drawing, painting, sculpting, or crafts in wood, plastics, metals, or leather are often used as therapies to relax highly stressed individuals. It can be tranquilizing to work with your hands or in any creative manner that switches your focus and lets you express your feelings without being dependent on words.

SINGING AND MUSIC: In general, these can elevate or soothe your feelings and even generate endorphins, depending on the music you select. Uninhibited singing is also a way of expressing your feelings, dissipating the negative emotions and elevating the positive feelings.

MEDITATION: This can be done in many different forms: through physical methods such as yoga, vocal methods such as chants, or mental methods such as counting your out breaths. Meditation requires a focus, such as a movement, a word, a color, a flickering candle. Listening to birds, wind chimes, music, or ocean sounds can facilitate meditation. Even listening to another person talk can be a type of meditation.

Biofeedback is Western meditation. A complex way to do it is by attaching yourself to equipment that measures a bodily function (brain waves, skin response, muscle tension, respiration) associated with the level of your stress or relaxation. It can be learned simply by taking your own pulse while you watch a clock.

BREATHING: Doing this in different ways can affect you differently depending on your needs. Slow, deep, rhythmic breaths without straining are most apt to be relaxing. Concentrate on breathing methods. Use all of your lungs gently and easily, and they become powerful relaxers.

JUGGLING OR BALANCING: These require intense concentration. To pause for even an instant means things fall apart. This is certainly not the deepest form of relaxation, but it brings an alert attention when over-stimulated senses cannot find a focus. It can also be fun and entertaining so you don't forget the child in you, that part of you that is the creative and imaginative problem solver. Juggling may be used as a transition step into more deeply relaxing states.

MASSAGE: Variations include reflexology, acupres-sure, rolfing, chiropractic, naprapathy, shiatsu. They are all forms of communicating and breaking down strained defense barriers through touch, which the largest organ of the body, the skin, needs for positive survival. These healing procedures and/or tactile expressions are ex-tremely relaxing and generate endorphins that help gen-erate positive, secure feelings. Even the person doing the touching will benefit by feeling more relaxed.

SEXUAL RELEASE: This is also a means to relax. A healthy body prepares to have a sexual encounter many times each day. If a person does not respond to this a few or more times each week, a tension will build, and it could be unconsciously acted out with inappropriate eat-ing. In the absence of a loving partner, fantasy and mas-turbation are normal, healthy substitutes. Because be-ing comfortable with one's own sexuality is important to a balanced, healthful life, counseling may be helpful, especially if fears, dysfunction, or discomfort exist.

IMAGERY: FANTASY, VISUALIZATIONS, DREAMS, IMPLOSIVE THERAPY, and PARADOXICAL INTENTION are used for projecting what may happen and for reflect-ing upon what did happen, letting you move emotions up or down. Your vision enables creativity, motivation, deal-ing with fears, wish fulfillments, and, ultimately, im-proved self-image. They are the key to your emotional harmony and, thus, to your very meaning/purpose. Books, teachers, classes, and your environment can all help you learn these skills, but only *practice* will bring mastery.

Implosive therapy invites into your mind the thoughts you have been straining to push out. Instead of distracting yourself from stressful ideas, invite them in. Exaggerate what upsets you until it is totally unrealistic. Once you have become comfortable with the worst in your mind, reality is much easier to confront.

Paradoxical intention works best with implosive therapy. In this case, strain to feel what you have been avoiding. If you strain to feel angry while looking in the mirror, you will laugh. If you strain to relax, you'll be tense and vice versa.

SLEEP: Restful sleep certainly helps reduce stress of physical fatigue or with recovery from illness or injury. Nutrition habits, anxieties, and dreams can determine how restful your sleep is. It's best not to eat for two to three hours before bedtime. Drugs, smoking, and illness also can interfere with sleep. Current research indicates that most people do much better on at least eight hours of sleep. But be careful. Sleep is sometimes overused to escape a threatening world (asthenic reaction).

SELF-HYPNOSIS: This, autogenic training, and autosuggestion depend on mental pictures, along with your verbal self-direction. Using well-learned induction techniques, you guide yourself into altered states of consciousness where you will accept suggestions that allow you to function with no distracting pressure. You will be able to do things you could do anyway if only you did not doubt yourself. Tapes, books, classes, and personal instruction from a psychologist can all result in mastery if you will *Practice! Practice! Practice!*

PROGRESSIVE MUSCLE RELAXATION: This is a simple method you can use anywhere, at any time, with no equipment. While seated or prone, close your eyes and visualize your feet. Contract the muscles in your feet tightly for five seconds and then suddenly relax your feet as you breathe gently. Next, focus on your calf muscles, repeating the process and isolating them from the muscles around them. It is the focus in your mind and the isolation of some muscles from the others that require the concentration that allows you to relax. Move from one muscle group to another with this process, tightening, holding, isolating, focusing, and relaxing as you go, while breathing in a gentle, easy, relaxed manner.

BIOENERGETICS: This is the release of emotional energy stored in your body. Screaming, yelling, hitting soft things, or physically acting out your feelings brings a release that allows for calmness. Professional assistance should be obtained when learning these methods.

AROMA THERAPY: Smell is not only the strongest of our memories but is also related to emotions (especially from childhood). Knowing which smells effect which emotions could be useful. One researcher learned the smell of spiced apples can decrease stress, increase alertness, reduce blood pressure, and wake up metabolism. Know your scents; use them where you need them.

SENSORY DEPRIVATION: This special technique is not suitable for everyone. It should only be used under the supervision of a trained professional for it could increase stress for some people. This method eliminates all stimuli. The client floats in a saline solution at body temperature in total darkness, total silence, and total stillness for an hour or more. The effect can be dramatic.

NUTRITION: Clearly, this can be very important in preventing distress and encouraging relaxation. Simply eating high amounts of complex carbohydrates will help you deal with physical/emotional aspects of stress. Staying away from refined sugars and food additives, especially caffeine, will also help you avoid distress symptoms. Remember, eating in response to stress wipes out any benefit of healthy eating as a form of stress reduction. When you are under stress, it is possible to develop deficiencies of B and C vitamins, calcium, or magnesium because the body uses them more rapidly, especially if you drink alcohol, smoke, or use certain drugs. Some supplements, such as niacin, can help, provided you don't have high blood pressure. Also, some herb teas, such as camomile, comfrey, or blends may add to a more relaxed mood. You should also seek professional advice from an herbalist, a nutritionist with a well-rounded background, or a physician who has acquired nutritional training beyond his or her medical program.

Remember that you are unique, and developing your *own* routines to deal with stress is a good idea. When learning techniques, you must be patient with yourself, forgiving when you get off track, non-critical when you make a mistake or are slow to learn, and encouraging with your self-talk. The relaxation method or methods that are most apt to be used well by you are the ones you believe will be helpful. The method "it" is not in question, but how you use it and feel about it make the difference.

Developing your consciousness of stress or distress and your level of confidence in dealing with them will make a difference in how many hugs you will continue to need from the refrigerator. It can also make the difference in opening or blocking your potential for joy, good relationships, health, and general success.

We need our emotions, and even some useful stress, to reach peak experiences in our lives; however, we don't need all the pitfalls that excess distress can cause.

By living a healthful lifestyle and learning to believe in yourself, you will be able to seek challenges in change and thrive on it instead of avoiding it. You will be able to overcome perfectionistic tendencies. When relaxed, you are at your best. Your intellect is sharper, your creativity is heightened, your humor is keen, your perspective is broader, your ability to be empathetic is expanded, and your usable energy is increased.

And most importantly, being relaxed is the only time you can truly get outside yourself and beyond your own emotional needs in order to be able to love another person fully and not to expect anything in return. The higher the priority you give to learning and using your ability to deal with your emotions, to be centered, balanced, calm, relaxed, tranquil, peaceful, and loving, the higher the quality of everything in all of your life will be.

CHAPTER 9

The Road to Self-Efficacy

Louise has been in one type of weight-loss group or another for 10 years. Some were as small as three or four members, and others were as large as 40 or 50. A few were more like a class where the "leader" was teaching, with limited input from the members, while other groups were open, with discussion topics decided by the members, and the "facilitator" was used as a resource who stepped in when the group was stuck. Many of the groups Louise participated in were task-oriented with clear goals and objectives, while others had a continuing theme but little structure. One group had no structure other than the stated intention of each group member to actively work on self-identified changes.

The many leaders and facilitators were as different from one another as were the group members in their education levels, credentials, experience, attitudes, personality traits, motives, income status, emotional stability, professional backgrounds, philosophical orientations (e.g., religious to parapsychological), age, and gender.

Some groups were very conservative; others were very liberal. Some groups stuck rigidly to topics such as diet and exercise, and others talked about any and all subjects. Some groups were very tightly bonded and the members were faithful to one another and their group

leaders. Others had a rapid turnover, and few friendships were developed.

If nothing else, Louise was knowledgeable about
weight-loss groups; she knew the role she would play in
them and how to manipulate each group session away
from her hidden concerns. She was the classic disillu-
sioned dieter.

For Louise, the various weight-loss groups had
served as entertainment; an escape from a house without love; a social network to develop friends; a place to
play and laugh; a distraction from her pain; and a place
to hide from her concerns while receiving emotional support and positive confirmation. The only thing Louise
really didn't like about the groups was the times a group
leader or facilitator would bring the group's attention to
bear on *her* and ask serious, confronting questions
about her feelings and thoughts. A number of times
Louise felt frightened when powerful emotions were ex-
pressed and horrifying stories were told or when group
members would get into a confrontation that couldn't
seem to be resolved.

But, overall, the groups *felt* like a positive experience to Louise and fulfilled many of her needs on a
short-term basis. The question was, did the groups serve
the purpose for which they were designed, or in any way
did personal growth or meaningful change result from
the many hours and money spent? Was Louise any better off for having attended them, or did the group only
provide entertaining procrastination?

The answers to these questions may be very subjective and difficult to assess; however, after examining
both the intended purposes of the group and Louise's
stated intention in joining them, a few answers appear to
be quite clear.

The groups didn't affect her relationship to her refrigerator. She did acquire much information, but she
didn't make any real, long-term effort to use any of it.
Education wasn't the same as application.

At this point, Louise feels that the unrestricted, unstructured weight-loss groups gave her the most insight into herself and to helping her understand why she wasn't using the information she had available to her. She still, however, cannot understand why she continued to procrastinate. She acknowledged using the groups for all the wrong reasons and feeling guilty at times for knowingly doing so without admitting it to others or, at times, even to herself.

When the last group ended, she knew she didn't want to seek another, and she felt a little lost and panicky about just what to do. She also felt sad and a little depressed, as though she had lost a good friend. Louise knew she could contact any of her old group members, but she also knew it would just be another way to procrastinate. She was frightened, but she didn't want to go back or hide any longer from changing her perfectionistic, people-pleaser, caretaker, co-dependent, non-assertive behavior. She didn't want to hide from her eating habits either. She just wasn't sure how to bring the changes about.

A New Group — A New Focus

It was a beautiful fall Saturday, and Louise was waiting for a friend across from a public park. As she sat in her car she noticed a group of people in the park doing an exercise together — an exercise she had learned about in the wellness program. The group completely captured her attention, and she quickly became enraptured with the beauty of the movements. Her busy, worried mind seemed to quiet down and do nothing more than focus on the movements. Louise realized a deep calm had come over her when her friend arrived, touched her, and asked if anything was wrong. It was a new and wonderful experience, and it was no surprise to find Louise a part of the exercise group the following Saturday.

Tai Chi Chuan is the exercise that attracted Louise. Louise valued it first as a way of quieting her mind and delivering the sense of peace she felt whenever she practiced, but it also gave her a feeling of connection with everything around her and a clarity in her thinking. If it had given her nothing else, she would have continued her training. She did not feel particularly skilled in Tai Chi, but as time went on, she developed her movements to the point where her teacher asked her to take part in a group demonstration.

This excited and frightened Louise at the same time. She practiced extremely hard in the days before the event. Then the day before her performance, she pulled a muscle in her back and was unable to take part in the demonstration. **Her teacher told her she was trying too hard to be the best (her old perfectionism getting in the way) and that she only needed to keep practicing her routines over and over to reach excellence and learn patience.** Louise wondered if she had subconsciously sabotaged herself as a way to avoid the pressure of possible failure.

Weeks passed, and her teacher did not ask her to take part in the next several demonstrations. Some days she felt like she was making little or no progress, and sometimes she didn't want to practice at all. She would go to practice anyway, go through the same familiar motions, and leave practice mellow and energetic and happy that she had taken part. Gradually, she forgot about the demonstrations, and except for a few missed practices, soon she had spent a year just going through the movements.

Then, after practice one Saturday, the teacher asked her if she would take part in a demonstration at a conference. She hadn't thought about it for so long it took her by surprise. She was also flattered and said she would. She remembered what her instructor had said: "Just stay with your usual routine."

This time it all came off beautifully. Louise knew she had reached a new level in her Tai Chi, but she also knew she had come to enjoy the *simple practice* more than reaching a recognized level of mastery. She knew if she were to reach still higher levels, they would come when she had put in much more time simply going through the basic movements and that pushing and straining to make it happen faster would only be counterproductive.

Mastering the Moment

Louise had discovered the important concept of mastery in the course of seeking her new group. Dr. George Leonard, author of *Mastery*, encourages us to live more fully in the present moment, to seek a natural rhythm instead of attempting to force, control, or contain behavior. His concept of mastery is more fully developed in the chapter on "Healthful Exercise." It is useful to find an activity with which you can realize the advantages of this focus. If disciplines, such as martial arts, meditation, or yoga are too esoteric or too difficult to identify with, try something closer to your current interests and values. Those activities that you believe add to your health bring with them additional psychological and motivational benefits and may serve you best.

Painting, knitting, dancing, carpentry, biking, gardening, public speaking, or playing an instrument are just a few examples of activities that can be used to work toward mastery of a discipline. **What is important is that you choose; that you allow yourself to be fully engrossed and consistent with what you choose; and that you approach it in such a manner that you don't try to control it but rather allow yourself to find harmony with it.**

When the Tai Chi experience came along, Louise had been out of her current weight-loss group for several weeks, and life was about the same as it had been before group. She did not feel as though she was looking for a substitute for the group; she had more or less let go of her weight struggle when she noticed the Tai Chi class in the park.

Louise does not believe she was drawn to Tai Chi for any of the old reasons that had formerly drawn her to all those group sessions. She had no role to play in Tai Chi as she had in her weight-loss groups. She had no ulterior motive for attending these classes. She was not even there for weight loss. She was there to experience the physical movement. Except on the occasions when her teacher asked her to help with a demonstration, she did not feel that she was "performing" for anyone. Her experience with Tai Chi wasn't like her aerobic weight-loss classes either, since neither she nor anybody else had any expectations for anything in particular to happen as a result of the class. Very little talking was done with other class members or by the teacher. It was mostly just practicing the movements over and over again. But there were benefits.

With the practice came calm, yet energetic feelings. Her moods improved, she felt better physically, her little nervous tics started to disappear, and even her back felt better. Her interest and attitudes about food were changing to the point where she noticed it, but she did not get excited about gradually losing a few pounds. Her focus stayed on the movement and satisfaction with the practice. The second time her teacher asked her to help with a demonstration, she realized that she had changed herself. Louise *felt* alive and more certain about what she could do. She felt she was in harmony with herself and her world, and what fears remained she knew she could deal with. Even realizing that life would never be perfect was liberating.

Now that Louise is *not* a part of a weight-loss group, she is functioning at a higher level of self-efficacy than at any time during or prior to attending groups. Judging solely by her statements and her appearance, it seems that she is more consistent with her diet, exercise, personal growth (assertiveness), and relaxation program (Tai Chi) now than in the past.

Yes, Louise was still in a group, but it was a very different group. The game was over, and she simply used the group as a means of channeling her efforts. She no longer focused on outcomes or social approval. She had allowed herself to look inside without intending to do so. Very little of what went on in class was intellectual or even verbal, yet her insights and understandings about herself seemed to be realized in a way they never had been before. **Louise was empowering herself through mastery. She was gaining self-esteem, harmony, and self-confidence, which made it easier for her to use her wellness lifestyle information.** She didn't go into the process with the intention of gaining harmony; it just seemed to come as an unexpected by-product of the practice.

Empowerment

Empowerment can be one result of working at mastery or something that is worked at in a more direct, cognitive manner. To empower yourself is to give yourself the means to achieve self-efficacy. Self-efficacy is the conviction that you can successfully change your behavior to reach your goals.

Empowerment, like mastery, is a method of changing your self-image and raising self-esteem, things that chronically overweight people tend to lose sight of in their impatient rush to lose weight.

Co-dependency therapists and business management consultants strongly promote the concept of empowerment, and even some political and school reform movements have adopted empowerment to raise self-esteem for children, parents, and to help employees to feel a sense of ownership with their jobs and life responsibilities. Compulsive behaviors can indicate the lack of empowerment attitudes.

Some of the practices involved in self-empowerment include:
- A COMMITMENT to stick with your vision through the easy and hard times is a must. This means a commitment that has such a high priority on your list of values that very few, if any, other values will supersede it. A clarity of exactly what the commitment includes is required so you won't ignore it in the midst of day-to-day distractions.

- A DISCIPLINE to follow through on the commitment is equally important, as shown in the way it served Louise. Also, it is extremely important to reach down deep for the courage inside when you don't think it is there and when you think your fear of staying on track is about to overwhelm you. Don't forget to give yourself credit (a mental pat on the back) when you are afraid to do something and you do it anyway.

- A RELATIONSHIP dedicated to supporting personal growth certainly contributed to the long-term success of the 5-Plus Club members. A friendship, a spouse, siblings, even kids for whom you are a role model, or professionals who also serve as friends can all be a part of the support with which you sustain your effort. Again, be very clear on exactly what is supportive to personal growth and how to adjust it when changes or good intentions have gone awry.

- SPONTANEITY AND INTUITION will serve you much better in the long run than having a structured plan devised for you. You need a sense of your body and what it needs — not just a calorie count to force yourself to stick to. A quick decision to get out of bed for that early morning jog rather than a long mental struggle about the pros and cons of getting started or staying in bed works better. Some decisions about where you want to go are not always clear or easy, and your gut-level intuition usually provides a good sense of what will work; learn to trust it. Practice being in touch with your feelings at the time you feel them. It will help immensely. So will knowing what you are telling yourself and imaging in your mind at any given moment.

- HUMOR AND PLAY can get you through the hard times and beyond your emotional burdens. Humor and play are natural, and whenever you are not too intense, you allow them to come out.

Humor and play are very practical when you think about it. Norman Cousins believes humor is what saved him from a terminal illness and a heart attack, and he has written several books on the subject. Most of all, humor and play help us to know we are alive and turn what could be depressing life and work situations into fun. They support the positive attitudes that lead to discovering our full potential to not only succeed but to thrive.

- NURTURING SELF-WORTH is essentially being responsible for yourself. It means taking enough of your own time, energy, thought, and other means to bring your health and well-being to a point where you realize the benefits of these priorities. You do this not only for your own physical and emotional well-being, but because you see that love, acceptance, and respect from others also come with it. In taking care of yourself, you also have a greater, wiser capacity when you do give to others. Nurturing self-worth often brings feelings of guilt until you start recognizing your own worth. Without going through this practice, all the other empowerment practices will be for naught.

- OWNERSHIP of responsibility for who and what you are as a person — the feelings you generate, the behaviors you choose, the beliefs you hold, and your responses to your life experiences — is empowerment. How you accept the ownership, be it with desire or trepidation, reluctance or enthusiasm, makes a great difference as to the satisfaction of ownership. It belongs to you; it always has and it always will — whether you want it or not, it's yours. To become what you want is your freedom or a huge burden to carry for life. It is where you have the best chance to thrive.

- ADJUSTING to the experiences of your life as they happen is necessary to finding harmony. Trying to stay the same while the world around you changes or as time and experience change what goes on within you is like trying to hold the river with your hands; you are overwhelmed or become so exhausted you simply let go and get pushed along. You don't stand still but are always moving forward or backward. For some people, the choice of learning to let go or relax is the first step forward.

- FULL-SPECTRUM PERSPECTIVE of your life and the world you live in is essential, especially in dealing with perfectionistic details. If you have full-spectrum perspective when looking at your flat tire on a hot day when you are dressed for an important appointment for which you are about to be late, you are able to see your life in total, that is, all you have lived and all you have left to live. In that moment, the situation can be seen as the *very small* part of your life that it is. With this perspective, you are able to handle problems better, recover from them more quickly, and even laugh about them later with a minimum of distress.

Empowerment, then, is the road to self-efficacy you always had before you that you now choose to take. It is an attitude and a way of viewing yourself and your world that allow the best of whatever you are to be realized. Like mastery, it brings you to a less conflicted and more harmonious, balanced center where extremes, such as obesity, don't exist.

Troubled Groups

In my earlier book, *Change Your Mind/Change Your Weight*, the chapter "Putting It All Together" includes a section on weight-loss support groups, and those pages are still true. It talks about how to select a weight-loss group, how to get the most out of the group, the way the group is intended to function, assessing the leader, your opportunity and responsibility to benefit from group, etc. What I now explain is why some weight-loss groups can work against you and give a clear explanation of what, in my opinion, is the most important aspect of a group: proactive change, where the group's culture fosters self-motivated change in the individual.

Problems with weight-loss groups often stem from the nature of the person leading them.

A group *leader* conducts group sessions. This take-charge person determines direction and topics, instructs members on how to correct their concerns, provides organization (structure), and usually will not risk confronting individuals for fear of being seen as unkind. A group leader will modestly accept praise (credit) for group or individual success and perceived personal growth or short-term weight loss and overlook regained weight.

In very subtle ways, possibly even unnoticed by the leader, the supportiveness of the group results in a bonding of the people who are a part of it, and gradually the group becomes dependent upon itself. Individuals believe that they cannot continue their short-term success on their own, and often, in fear of losing the group, turn to the leader to save them. The leader, blinded by his or her own ego needs, revels in the flattery, assumes the protective parent role, and rescues the fearful members who are still full of self-doubt, possibly after months or even years of attending the group.

No individual is really at fault in this situation, including the group leader. This type of group usually has a clear goal of getting the weight off while providing emotional support along with an understanding of how the problem came about and behavioral means of resolving it.

The group dependency comes about because the co-dependent personalities come together with their care-taker/people-pleasing skills in full force. They like one another for that reason, sharing and laughing in a way they usually don't at home or work and having a leader who needs approval and praise as much as anyone in the group. Analyzing their concerns and seeking answers with the group and leader quickly seem comfortable. Receiving praise and approval from the group for small changes and comforting reassurance for slips in their organized plan make the usual critical self-talk go away for a while. The co-dependent group becomes like an extended family to hang on to for a while.

Things usually start falling apart within three to six months thereafter. Many of the participants who don't lose much weight early in the program drop out. Others who have lost weight start to regain it and are embarrassed to return to group. A smaller number of hard-core members will stay with the leader, many times for years, and add or continue individual counseling with the leader.

Popularity, new dependencies, avoiding discomfort, entertainment, extended families, ongoing psychoanalysis 101, and "guruitis" were never what anybody intended the weight-loss group to provide. It happens because individual group members and the group as a whole are avoiding risk, challenge, or fear, or the program is being perpetuated for financial reasons or the leader's ego needs.

Weight-loss groups, other than those that promote products or services as saviors, most often are well intended. As a rule, the group or program includes simple, infantilizing (you're not bright enough to figure it out yourself) behavioral methods that are stressed over and over. This certainly relieves the overweight person of making decisions, learning to believe in himself or herself, and taking responsibility for the long-term outcome. Short-term credit always goes to the product, service, or leader. When weight is regained, blame is placed upon the group member for not staying with the rules, on problems at home, or on the outside world, but never on the design of the group.

However, you should not conclude that groups are categorically bad. They can sometimes help you. But you must be cautious and have your own goals and expectations, as I suggest below.

Proactive Change

Proactive change involves gradual, self-initiated personal development activities (change through risk-taking). You use your own fears, questions, and problems to strengthen your self-image through the use of intellectual, social, and physical challenges. The objective is not only personal change that is wellness-oriented and holistic but also discovery of new, self-enhancing potentials.

If you are seeking a weight-loss group, consider one that follows Dr. Albert Ellis's philosophy of rational-emotive therapy. This is a technique of learning to anticipate and understand emotional responses, especially to stressful stimuli. Importantly, it fosters the belief that you can choose your behaviors and change them as necessary. A weight-loss group that follows this philosophy is one that will help create proactive change in you.

Challenges

The following challenges are typical of what you should expect to initiate from a proactive-change weight-loss group. If you are not finding these kinds of activities in your weight-loss group, or being sparked by your group, consider suggesting them, or go ahead and try them on your own.

The challenges are at three levels of difficulty. You complete the first series within the group setting. The second series you complete outside of the group but together with one or more supportive individuals. You complete the last and most difficult series on your own. Modify and adapt this suggested list to meet your individual needs or use it as a basis for creative efforts by the members in your weight-loss group to design and plan their own.

You determine the degree of risk in each activity. What may be difficult for one member may be very easy for you. The idea is to always be in a process of identifying, planning, confronting, relating, or adjusting challenges to be faced, advancing to more difficult challenges as your confidence grows. Keeping activities frequent will speed up ever-developing self-esteem. Any challenge that is resolved will affect your ability to better deal with matters of choice, such as diet and exercise.

To be fearful is an opportunity to know your courage. Because every activity is self-initiated, honest, open sharing is essential to personal success. Only you can know for sure how much of a risk you are taking, but most other people who know you will notice changes in self-esteem, image, trust, confidence, and belief if you have taken true risks.

Proactive risk-taking is not meant for entertainment or thrills. It is meant to be done with serious intent, planning, and care. The purpose is to improve your self-image, self-trust, and confidence. The main fears common to all humans are:

- Fear of pain (physical and emotional).
- Fear of embarrassment.
- Fear of losing what we have.
- Fear of not getting what we want.
- Fear of fear.

Listen to your body, which expresses your emotions and you'll know when you are out of your comfort zone and close to your fears. Once you become aware of discomfort (fear), the risk is in confronting it. A good book on risk-taking is *Risk-Taking for Personal Growth* by Joseph Ilardo, Ph.D.

Series I Challenges

The following challenges (risks) are meant to be done within your weight-loss group setting. You should design your own challenge, the time to confront it, and whether you will do it alone or with other members.

- Complete your philosophy-of-life organizer and value priorities list.
- Lead the group in a self-improvement exercise using details from a group exercise guide or a self-created plan.

- Do a reading or act out a scene that takes you out of the character type people know you by.
- Sing a song that expresses some strong feelings either to the group or one individual in the group.
- Give a serious, prepared ten-minute talk that supports an idea you are very much against.
- Tell two group members what you believe would make them more successful and popular.
- Do a dance that tells your story of fears and hopes.
- Do five minutes of stand-up comedy.
- Express yourself for three minutes without protecting your self-image in any way, that is, be fully yourself.
- Communicate your feelings non-verbally to another group member or to the full group for five minutes.
- Share a creative idea or poem you've written with the group.

Series II Challenges

You should do the following challenges (risks) outside of the group setting with another group member or person of your choice. All aspects of the proactive group will still apply. You are in charge of knowing when you are out of your comfort zone or if you should withdraw to prepare for a later attempt. It is not necessary to put your personal safety in jeopardy to achieve your goal. Just getting on stage makes you a success. The following menu of activities is only to stimulate your own imagination. You can pick from the menu if you like, modify something from the menu, or create something special. Keep in mind that time for careful planning is one thing, procrastination is another.

- Spend a day working at a food kitchen for the homeless.

- Go for a sailplane ride or take an introductory flying lesson.
- Conduct a survey at the airport of at least 20 people.
- Caddy for strangers at a golf course.
- Put on a bring-one-person-you'd-like-to-meet party.
- Put on a new-games party for families, with no food.
- Climb to a peak that is higher than you've ever been.
- Apply for a job for which you have no experience and/or for which you have no interest.
- Ride the city bus as far as you can on a single ticket.
- Create a healthful (non-fattening) dish and try to have it put on the menu of a local cafe.
- Change your hairstyle dramatically.
- Develop a completely different clothing outfit that is a departure from your usual style of dress.

Series III Challenges

The following challenges are meant to be done by you *independently*. All aspects of the proactive group still apply. You are still in charge of knowing when you are out of your comfort zone and if you should withdraw to prepare for another attempt. If your personal safety is in jeopardy, your first priority is to reevaluate your path to your goals and take a less precarious road. You are still able to pick from the menu, modify a menu choice, or create your own challenge to fit your needs. Remember, the closer you experience challenges, the sooner the changed view of yourself will come about.

- Spend a Sunday visiting with the elderly in a nursing home.
- Make a gift and give it to a person you care about when it isn't a special occasion.

- Spend a day in stores, offices, and cafes, and meet at least eight people. Find out what they are afraid of.
- Meet with authorities from religion, art, law, and education and ask an open-ended question such as: "Why can't people get along?"
- Put yourself in various situations where you tend to be impatient, and while you are waiting, try to figure out why you are so impatient.
- Spend a weekend alone in a cabin, camping, or any place you can be without books, radio, TV, or other distractions.
- Arrange to ride in a police car for several hours one evening.
- Arrange to do cold-call selling one full day.

Monitoring your own feelings and setting up your own challenges will undoubtedly serve you the best. A proactive group well used will serve as an initial base and a means of channeling your efforts as well as a launching pad for future efforts on your own. If you find yourself in a weight-loss group where new insights are no longer being acquired and where you are not initiating your own new efforts, it is very possible you are in group for the wrong reasons.

Group support is not for everybody with a weight problem, or it may not be for the long term. **If you are not growing beyond the need for the group, the group may be more for the benefit of those who set it up. Whatever the group is, remember it is not going to change you. You are going to change you. Self-change is the change that lasts.**

If you think you could benefit from group participation, consider all types before you decide which is right for you. Depending on your situation, a toastmasters club or tennis club may be more valuable to you than a dedicated weight-loss group. Last, but not least, try to gather some statistics on the long-term benefits of any group you are considering. Determine the philosophy, personality, intention, and needs of the group leader. If you can clearly see within a few weeks that you are not making good use of a group, it would seem time for reevaluation or departure. Similarly, though you may find benefits from being part of a weight-loss group, make sure the benefits are continuing, that you haven't outgrown the group. The biggest danger to weight-loss groups is that they can provide a rationalization for procrastinating. And there is an alternative.

CHAPTER 10

Procrastination to Motivation

We are motivated to inaction just as we are motivated to action. If we procrastinate, we have a reason for putting off something we think we *want* to do, something we *should* do, or something we *have* to do in favor of other motivations.

Chronic procrastination is not just a bad habit but a way of expressing internal conflict and protecting a vulnerable sense of self-esteem. Often this is a direct result of perfectionistic attitudes. If it can't be done exactly right, or if there is a possibility of failure, the perfectionist will postpone the initiative. Few people give up procrastinating until they understand the function it serves in their lives. They also need to know why their self-esteem is low and how putting things off acts as a buffer for their shaky sense of self-worth. Learning to find the energy and courage to get beyond procrastination is, of course, the beginning of changing this defense mechanism that puts too many limits on the potential of an exciting life.

Chronic procrastinators are not lazy people. Moralizing and labeling them as lacking ambition or discipline only reinforce the sense of inadequacy and become self-fulfilling prophecies. I also do not believe that chronic procrastination is merely a lack of organization.

Where consistent, long-term behavior is concerned, such as with weight loss, organization may only add to the problem. Remember that people who are successful in losing weight and keeping it off over the long term and who are comfortable with their behavior achieve their success through spontaneity rather than through plans, structure, organization, or control. At some point, everyone procrastinates. How frequently and regarding how many different matters vary from person to person. Sometimes we are very much aware of why we procrastinate, sometimes we do not wish to know, and sometimes it is just puzzling to us.

Procrastination as it relates to weight loss is one of those puzzling times.

Louise felt she had explored the depths of her soul, and I know we attempted to explore the depths of her mind, trying to discover why she did not do what she was so certain she wanted to do.

"If you consider the thousands of dollars, the time, and the energy I've spent trying to get the pounds off, isn't that proof that I really want to be thin?" she would say with great emotional pain.

Louise and I considered many possible motives for her procrastination about losing weight. One of the things Louise procrastinated about was making a decision about which of many possible motives was at the core of her procrastination. All the reasons sounded plausible to Louise, just as they can for anyone wanting to lose weight yet not doing so.

There are several common "reasons" for not losing weight.

- You won't know for sure if your spouse loves you only for your body.
- You would be giving in to your spouse's control.
- You would become promiscuous because you would be more sexually attractive.
- You would no longer have an excuse for avoiding difficult challenges.

- You would lose attention and sympathy for your unsuccessful weight-loss attempts.
- You would lose a part of your identity.
- You would lose your excuse for falling short of your goals.
- You would lose your power to manipulate family and friends.
- You would lose some of your "friends" because of your success.
- You would have no means (food) of rewarding yourself.
- You would lose your means of diminishing anxiety with the comfort of food.
- You would lose your means (food) of achieving pleasure.
- You would lose your means of relieving frustration and feelings of deprivation.
- You would lose your means of expressing your hostility.
- You would lose your means of diminishing your insecurity.
- You would lose your means of self-punishment to soothe your guilt.
- You would lose your means of proving your own inferiority.
- You would find it harder to avoid change.

If one or all of these motives were true, it could be enough for Louise to procrastinate about her weight loss. But Louise always felt that something still deeper, something in her subconscious, was really at the root of why she remained overweight. Perhaps, she thought, at the root of her procrastination was a trauma she had experienced as a child that was too horrible to recall.

Louise wanted to believe it was something *beyond her control* or something she knew nothing about, something that would relieve her of the responsibility to do anything. Without knowing "for sure" what was wrong, avoiding the risk of failure was certainly justified in her thinking.

Louise, like so many others, was bright and able to rationalize. She was able to create reasons not to follow through with her plans; to find ample cause to avoid her fears; and to look like a martyr, a caring mother, a loyal friend, and a selfless person who always put the needs of others ahead of "her own."

Many theorists lean heavily on oral fixations learned in the childhood experience of bonding with their primary security/love object during feeding and to underfeeding or overfeeding in response to the cries of the child regardless of the hunger need. It does happen that overprotective parents and "busy" parents often use food to deal with all the child's emotional needs, as a cure for boredom, or to express love. ("Nothin says lovin' like somethin' from the oven.") As the child develops, the line between physical hunger and emotional needs becomes blurred. **Eventually, hunger pangs may not be recognized at all by the overweight person because all the other stimuli that are responded to with eating seldom leave time for the hunger need to develop.**

For Louise, the blur of possible motivations to eat inappropriately and stay overweight cleared up as she calmed herself.

By mastering Tai Chi, she became more focused and, thus, was more often calm. When we are relaxed, at peace with ourselves, and feeling safe, we see ourselves more clearly and sense our emotions, drives, and intuitions more accurately. Tai Chi provided this for Louise, but it could just as easily be something else for another person.

As Louise stayed calm for longer periods of time, her need to eat inappropriately grew less until she actually felt true hunger pangs again. Because her ability to focus and sense her feelings had improved a great deal, she realized what was happening within herself. Louise also realized that her strongest drive was for affiliation, the need to feel close to, loved, and accepted by important people in her life.

Because she came to feel more safe in her adult world, she was also able to recall events that had taken place with her father when she was a child. Mostly the fears were regarding possible physical abuse and abandonment threatened by her drunken father. When drunk, he would state these threats so graphically that Louise could not bear the thought of them. By feeling safe in her world today, Louise was able to open the door for these powerful, overwhelming memories to come to the surface of her consciousness.

Some methods for exploring subconscious motives are hypnosis; tests, such as the Thematic Apperception Test (TAT); psychotherapy; and the best method, through well-practiced relaxation techniques. The point here is that only Louise could know the answers for sure; the rest was all speculation, analysis, and guesswork. Some of that analysis was correct but never provable or complete until Louise was ready to reexperience her deeper fears.

Knowing why people hang on to the habits that keep them overweight doesn't necessarily mean the behavior will change, but the new-found certainty of what needs to be dealt with makes denial difficult, and procrastination becomes more uncomfortable. Understanding our motives can be very confusing when they are tied into our past experiences, ever-changing circumstances, and the emotions that we have been conditioned with from childhood.

A great deal of the process Louise went through to understand herself and avoid her fears was part of the learning process necessary to a full understanding and clear perception of herself. The only qualification was that the whole process of finding her way did not need to take nearly so long. Many of the commercial programs, diets, and gurus had served more as distractions and escapes without which Louise could have succeeded much faster.

The Cost of Procrastination

The cost of procrastination for the seriously over-weight person is very high. Even though it may seem easier to avoid fears than to confront them, the prices paid in the long run are much greater if we procrastinate. Here are some of the costs of procrastination.

- EMOTIONAL PAIN: Guilt results from knowing what "should" be done, fear of what others will think, and embarrassment when others know. Anxiety, depression, loneliness, obsessive-compulsiveness, and even suicide may occur in this circle of self-defeating behavior.
- LOW SELF-ESTEEM: We tend to believe about ourselves what we see ourselves do. Chronic procrastination leads us to believe we are incapable, undependable, undeserving, inadequate, and unloveable.
- LOST OPPORTUNITIES: Achievement, money, relationships, a sense of aliveness, and meaning or purpose may all slip by the procrastinator, but worst of all, the opportunity to like, trust, and believe in yourself is lost by not deciding to take action that works.
- DECREASED PRODUCTIVITY: Without action, fewer goals are achieved in most areas of life. The procrastinator then believes he or she is a failure, feels depressed, and has little energy to try the next time, which means more procrastination. Logically, of course, putting efforts off and postponing needs always get less done.
- TROUBLED RELATIONSHIPS: Significant others lose respect, trust, and confidence in the procrastinator. Procrastinators are often perfectionistic, critical, easily upset, hurt, disappointed, angered, and worst of all, fearful, meaning the "real" person is not seen, making them very difficult to like or get along with.
- IMPAIRED HEALTH: Procrastinators are more easily distressed, and distress leads to illness.

Putting off the activities of a healthful lifestyle may mean continued obesity, a weakened heart, high blood fat, more colds and ailments of all kinds, not to mention emotional disorders like depression, anxiety, and serious mood disorders.

- LOSS OF TIME: Procrastination often means killing life's most precious commodity — the time we have to live — by waiting for conditions to improve; waiting for our fears to vanish; doing busy work to distract attention from what is important; and missing fulfillment by living in the past, future, or fantasies. Not being in the "moment" is putting off the opportunities to experience joy, happiness, and enhancing self-worth with a sense of being alive — all of which are found only on the edge of the comfort zone.

It is clear that procrastination is not an intellectual matter but rather an emotional one. The cost of procrastination is too high to be a choice of logic or reason. Bright procrastinators, however, are very able to convince themselves that their procrastination makes sense and serves a purpose. We can cleverly tie our postponements to other, "selfless" values. Who can point a finger of blame when our reasons for procrastination are for the job (family income), our friend, the spouse, or a parent and not "just" a selfish need of our own? Procrastination can help us to avoid the fears of success, guilt, new challenges, etc. But it also can provide us with the rewards or secondary gains of revenge, power, and rebellion, etc., to which we may not want to admit.

To find overriding motivations for those reasons we use to justify our procrastination and then to rearrange our value priorities is to realize that motivation builds on itself. Enabling ourselves usually takes more than one insight, one event, or one person; it takes a whole series of self-initiated actions done with some regularity. But it can be done.

Letting Go of Procrastination

It is not important that you stick to this entire list of suggestions or that you follow them in any specific order. What is important is that you keep the action going, that you are sincere and realistic with your efforts, and that you are willing to take some risks, knowing that most of your efforts will pay off if you do not overwhelm yourself with your expectations and are willing to get up and try again when you fall down. Choose one or two of these suggestions and give them an open-minded trial. Some will appeal to you, others may not. Choose those that best fit your circumstances.

- Monitor your self-talk to notice the mental struggles (conflict) going on over what you logically believe (e.g., eating healthy) and what you emotionally want (e.g., fattening foods). Learn how to quiet your mind through some practice like meditation, yoga, or Tai Chi. If you follow through on any of these tips, the mental struggle about what you are choosing to eat will stop.

- Listen to your body to learn of your fears. Instead of avoiding your fears, gradually and deliberately go toward your fears to desensitize yourself and learn that you are able to resolve them. From this behavior you learn to trust yourself and reduce your need to procrastinate.

- Confront your guilt feelings by practicing "active forgiveness." Take time usually given to being responsible *for* others and use it being responsible *to* others. This means being the model for others instead of the servant for others. Set the example of becoming healthy, happy, fulfilled, and liking the person you are.

- Stop blaming yourself for your imperfections. This will take you a long way toward being less angry and thus diminish some of the need to be overweight.

- Be willing to take some measured risks into the unknown with the awareness that some efforts will not pay off the first, second, or even third try. Both negative and positive risks in changing can be scary. Choose the ones that you can like yourself for even if they don't pay off in the way you had originally intended.

- Avoid analyzing and judging the meanings and feelings of others. Learn to inquire and listen with an open mind; listen without judgment, analysis, or preparing a response, and notice the payoff.

- Track your emotions with a daily log of events and your reactions to them. Ask yourself many times each day, "What am I feeling?" Then listen to your body for the answers. Notice how increased self-awareness improves your decisions and disposition.

- Keep things in perspective. Each time you realize you are emotionally upset, ask yourself five times quickly, "What does this mean in relation to my whole life?"

Notice that each suggestion to reduce procrastination requires action and some sort of consistent effort to follow through or change. These suggestions, like any number of others, can be something more to procrastinate about. The difference between these activities and those that have been procrastinated about is only the purpose; otherwise they are identical. Therefore, unless you have an extremely strong drive to become a non-procrastinator or have strong motivation to follow these tips for other reasons, it is unlikely the tips will be of great help. No matter what the action is or what is being avoided, if the procrastinating behavior is to change, motivation is the key needed.

Motivation Inside and Out

Where does motivation come from? Are we born with it like intelligence — some people with more, some with less? Is it something we learn from our environment? Can we learn to have more of it, especially about important needs we have? The answers may be uncertain, but

the truth of the matter is that people change from procrastinating to taking action every day, and it seems we
all have the ability to do it.

No doubt, if you are over 18, you have probably seen
yourself stop your procrastination and become a regular
doer of at least one thing you had previously avoided. A
few examples are learning to dance even though you
thought you had two left feet, giving up footballs for
dresses, flossing your teeth daily, voting, wearing a seat
belt, organizing your tax papers, exercising, or changing
an attitude about school, religion, marriage, parents.

Some of the things that you quit putting off you
actually learned to like, and some of them you waste
great amounts of emotional energy disliking but go right
on doing anyway. No matter what it was you stopped
postponing and started doing regularly, you created a
drive, a reason, a purpose, and a motivation (or many
motivations) to get yourself to do it. You wanted something more; you feared something more; you feared
something less; you understood a consequence better;
you paid the price for procrastinating one too many
times; your longing became overwhelming; you hurt too
badly physically or emotionally; it was the only socially
acceptable thing to do; or you simply came to realize you
could change, and it made sense to do so. In any case,
there was a possible payoff, benefit, reward, or punish-
ment of some kind that helped to bring about the
change.

**If we do not have enough motivation or motiva-
tors to stimulate action, we tend to look for ways to
make change easier.** The commercial weight-loss programs want to appear to be the ticket. The programs,
products, or services promise to require less effort (i.e.,
drive or motivation) from us so we do not have to rearrange our motivation priorities. The motivations to lose
weight do not have to be strong enough to override any
of the existing fears or rewards. The idea is that we hope
to have our cake and eat it too.

External motivators (such as commercial weight-loss schemes) are an excuse to procrastinate about learning to develop better intrinsic motivation skills. Most of us know that changing in order to please family, friends, or a spouse does not result in lasting changes. Even most weight-loss programs talk about doing it for yourself. It is easy to repeat this statement and believe we mean it. **Yet most of the motivation from any weight-loss program is intended to be external.** You need to look clearly at just whom it is you want to have feel better. Will you put your personal health care ahead of your job requirements five to 10 hours each week? Do you want so much to live to see your kids grow up that you will change the family menu?

Chronically overweight people are so used to putting perceived demands of others ahead of their own needs that it is hard for them to know what is for them and what is for others. It is also hard for this same group to understand just what a motivation to take care of themselves is all about.

When asked the question, "What does doing for yourself mean?" people most commonly answered: when I take bubble baths, buy myself some new clothes, or do less housework. Seldom is "doing for yourself" seen as action leading to having a healthier mind or body or "making decisions based on personal values and needs" seen as leading to greater self-esteem. Rest and escape activities are useful, but how is a person going to develop the self-efficacy that is missing by taking a bubble bath? In fact, lazing in a bath can be used to validate one's poor self-image, create guilt feelings, and promote a need for more sensual comforting in the form of food.

To chronically overweight people, reaching for external support seems easier and safer than the development of self-efficacy. They know many fewer decisions have to be made, meaning fewer mistakes are possible, and someone or something is available to blame if things do not work out. Why struggle with the risks of learning to motivate from within? Staying with external motivation (commercial help) and going with an easier way to get the job done are strong messages to the self not to trust or believe in that self.

In my last book, *Change Your Mind/Change Your Weight*, I spoke of the path to self-motivation that starts with desire, an element that may be lacking in a depressed person. Even if this most basic element is missing, it is usually temporary. Because we have eyes, ears, and a brain that is able to imagine in response to the stimuli of the environment, we are vulnerable to new possibilities that quickly retrieve desire or establish it anew. When we want something, we are open to seeing possibilities. Once we can see possibilities, we begin to see how we might attain our goal. We can take something that is possible and see it as probable, and this creates hope. When we hope, we can sense our goal within our reach. **Now how do we make that last step to get a hold of what we are after?**

At this point, we are still in an action phase, and this is where the individual effort may break down. This occurs just before we get to the top of the hill. External motivation has provided the power up to this point, except for the initial desire.

Remember that what we are after is a change in our own behavior. People often get this confused with thinking they need to focus on loss of pounds rather than on the attitudes and beliefs that lead to the behavior changes that will result in the loss of the pounds. If the focus of what we are trying to get (a lasting change in certain behaviors and ultimately a more self-efficacious view of ourselves) is not kept clear, we will get into trouble at this point. Also, if our motivation does not become an internal drive but rather remains external (e.g., commercial weight-loss programs, services, gurus, products, etc.), we will quickly be right back at the starting point of desire.

With an internal focus to gain greater self-awareness and clarity of one's own beliefs and value priorities, decisions are simpler and personal freedom is accepted.

If we accept that we are free to be who we want to be, it's much harder to find excuses and place blame for not changing. The difficulty is finding the courage to take the risks inherent in actively, deliberately, and consciously changing.

If we are clear about our goals, if we are self-efficacious, we are more likely to choose foods that will help us in our weight-loss effort. If our goal is before us, we can see what change in our daily routine will allow room for a regular exercise period.

Once the action of change has been experienced on a continuum, we tend to believe what we have seen ourselves do. Watching ourselves take the action and risk and achieve periodic gains, we come to believe we can count on ourselves to come through. Self-confidence and self-trust grow, and we are less likely to procrastinate about the next effort. Better yet, we realize we don't need to look to an outside provider for motivation.

Again, the answer lies in the problem. What we avoid doing because it is hard or we fear we will fail at doing is the very thing that can change our perception of ourselves and thus our inaction to action.

Motivation Systems

Dr. David McClelland, a Harvard professor who has researched motivation for more than 40 years, provides many insights in his book, *Human Motivation*. He indicates a clear element of subconscious motivation in all humans, including people like Louise, but he also talks of research that shows that we are aware of most of our motives.

Dr. McClelland speaks of four major motive systems: achievement, doing or gaining things we see as worthy; power, the ability to control our circumstances; affiliative, being loved and accepted; and avoidance, not having to face something undesirable. All seem to be tied into the understanding of the chronically overweight person. So many different aspects seem to influence motivation, from smell and taste memories or sex to unlimited factors of social environmental conditioning, that even with a high degree of self-awareness, most of us do not tie to our immediate urges each day all the different motivational factors and what influences them. **Understanding why we procrastinate about exercising or why we feel a need to eat when our stomach is already full requires a truly involved effort.** We must determine our stronger, basic underlying drives and explore our ever-shifting motivations and our ever-shifting experiences and environmental influences.

Confused? Who wouldn't be? The more one becomes involved with the academic research, the different theories, the means of measuring motivation, and the bringing together of the multiple variables of multiple personal motivations, the more confusing it can become. Reading or counseling with professionals who are able to be objective may be helpful in speeding up the process; however, each of us must determine the ultimate truth of why we don't do what seems logical or why we do what is often self-defeating in our own lives.

We do have similarities with certain groups of people who practice behaviors similar to our own, and we can learn from them as discussed earlier in this book with the 5-Plus Club. However, we are still unique individuals with unique circumstances that are constantly changing. The best part is that we are all existential beings with a large degree of free choice to influence our lives, which includes our motivations.

Learning how we can best motivate ourselves through our own insights into ourselves and the practice of those elements that give our lives a degree of peace, health, and self-efficacy certainly will lead to a life that is full, stimulating, satisfying, and an adventure that includes more harmony than discord. Excessive fat is a scarce commodity in a life that is intrinsically motivated.

CHAPTER 11

Changing Your Food Preferences

Louise laughed and blushed when I first asked her if she had ever been on a weight-loss diet before. She had tried *all* the popular diets over the years, at least for a few days. Some of them, such as Weight Watchers, she tried several times. She attempted a water fast, a liquid protein fast, the Atkins Diet, and the high-fiber diet. But the only time she had stayed with a reducing diet long enough to even come close to her ideal weight was when she took diet pills prescribed by a doctor.

Even during the years she was enrolled in my wellness weight-loss program, she used several extreme diets, such as the grapefruit, rice, and rotation diets. Louise had a collection of diet books larger than my own. In addition to the information Louise had gained from her extensive library, she had taken several correspondence courses in nutrition and had attended many nutrition workshops. Louise has a broad knowledge of nutrition, acquired from many "authorities" on the subject. Whenever she thinks of going back to college, it is always to become a registered dietitian. Even though each new weight-loss diet plan would come to the same end as the ones before it, Louise was still ready to optimistically embrace the next variation.

Whenever we spoke of the unlikely possibility that any "weight-loss" diet could change her behavior, she was in intellectual agreement. Emotionally, however, she would still cling to the hope that somehow the right diet combinations, timed right, with the right taste, volume, and variety would come along. And then, when she had found this magic combination so she wouldn't feel like she was on a diet, the "magic" would work, and she would become thin.

Midway through our work together, **Louise realized that just getting the weight off would not assure her of keeping it off**, so she gave up pursuing the rapid weight-loss methods. She also decided that in spite of some genetic heritage, her social and cultural conditioning, and the always present easy access to tempting fattening foods, it would still be possible for her to lose weight.

Having plenty of good information on healthful and non-fattening food, and letting go of the need for quick weight loss and all the old excuses for easy weight gain, Louise had moved herself further along the path of meaningful change to long-term success.

In a survey in the June 1993 issue of *Consumer Reports,* there are clear indications that not only Louise, but also many other Americans are becoming dissatisfied with diet fads. Crash diet programs are losing much of their old appeal. Getting rid of fat, junk foods, and protein fasting powders in favor of fruits and vegetables seems to be the new direction. As a society, we finally seem to be acknowledging that complex carbohydrates not only do not cause weight gain, but they actually help us a great deal, especially if we exercise in a reasonable manner.

Unlike Louise, many people don't have all the latest information regarding nutrition and weight loss. New, relevant information is bombarding us at such a rapid pace that it is difficult for specialists in the field, let alone the average person, to keep up.

Studies, such as those by Dr. Colin Campbell of Cornell University, have been going on for years. One of Dr. Campbell's many interesting findings is that, while eating substantially more calories than the average over-weight American, Chinese people in certain geographic areas do not develop weight problems. These people eat a low-fat, high-carbohydrate diet from local foods that are not processed or packaged. This finding indicates that it is not the *number* of calories, but the *type* of calories that makes the difference with weight problems. Campbell's China study is discussed in more detail later in this chapter.

We now know that all weight-loss diets are the wrong approach to weight loss, and to focus on them, even as a temporary solution, is counterproductive. Any very low-calorie diet is apt to end up causing problems rather than providing solutions. Some of the problems are potentially fatal.

The only weight-loss program that really has an excellent chance of working is a program developed by the individual using the basics that are focused on health. These should be choices that are comprehensive in scope, done without fanfare or special products, and that allow changes to come about slowly as the individual learns to prefer new healthful tastes and make positive food choices.

In this chapter, I have put those ideas into a system from which you can build your eating program. I know if you try to control your eating behavior through a plan structured by someone else, you will rebel eventually. Worse, you will not be building the much-needed self-confidence to be able to take charge of yourself and your own eating habits.

In recent years I have come to be certain about my belief in a vegetarian diet and that the closer you come to eating a vegan (no animal products) vegetarian diet, the healthier you will be and the less likely to encounter weight problems.

I have been a vegetarian since 1976, with all the benefits and inconveniences that entails. But, as I've often said to Louise, I don't recommend that anyone suddenly and dramatically take up this lifestyle for they are likely to burn out on it quickly. I also know that an overweight person can become trim without becoming a vegetarian. To me, however, it is the best way for the overweight person to gradually become healthy and slim.

Louise found the idea of becoming a vegan vegetarian somewhat overwhelming, but she had also come to realize that extreme weight-loss diets such as those she had tried are also very hard to live with. Now she has accepted the idea of building her own diet over a long period of time, and it is coming more easily. She has taken many of her old recipes for fattening foods and modified them with healthful ingredients. No control or dependency is involved. In her path to change she is learning to relax and find harmony between the emotions she creates in her mind and her knowledge and sense of her own body and what it needs.

Her struggle within herself and the parent/child struggles with the weight-loss authorities have ended. She has only the mild fear of change and her own impatience with which to deal. Like Louise, if you see the following food choice system as only one resource from which to build your own diet, though it may take some time and seem difficult now and then, you will be much more willing to accept your own changes and give yourself the credit you deserve for making self-directed changes.

Other resources for building healthful diets are all around you. The trick is to seek them out as you need them. Specialists in the field love to be asked questions, but you are responsible for asking and for what you do with the information.

Weight-loss diets have contributed far more to fat gains than to long-term fat losses for millions of people struggling to master their corpulence. Counting calories has proven to be aversive, and structured weight-loss diets deny individual free choices (taking charge of yourself). Nor do they allow for hour-to-hour, day-to-day changes in one's nutritional needs. If you are ever going to prefer healthful foods, enjoy their tastes, expand the variety of foods you eat, and have ample volume to satisfy your hunger and nutritional needs, changes will have to come not only from your environment but also from within you.

Changes in your attitudes are essential (e.g., "I can never like green stuff"), value priorities (e.g., "I always stay up to watch late-night TV and I'm too tired to get up early enough to exercise before going to work"), and your perception of your ability to eat in your own best interest (e.g., "I'll always prefer a good steak to a salad, and I'll always need some help to control my eating!").

Highly structured weight-loss diets are infantilizing and take away from your reasons to believe in yourself. Worse, weight-loss diets set up a control and dependency factor against which to rebel (e.g., "I was bad yesterday. I cheated on my diet, ha ha!"). Weight-loss diets imply that you are somehow inadequate and that you are not intelligent enough to make your own logical choices.

The real goal is for you to be able, with confidence, to make informed, independent, spontaneous decisions about what you eat, knowing the food will fill you, satisfy you, meet your nutritional needs, and taste good. You don't need mighty stores of willpower to force and control yourself in a struggle that will exhaust and defeat you in the end. Nor do you need a Ph.D. in nutrition. Simply take yourself through the following steps with the courage and sense of adventure you've always had but may have been afraid or reluctant to use.

Clarify Your Goals

Changing the volume, quality, and frequency of what you eat is highly important, but it is not nearly as important as changing your beliefs about your ability to change to healthful food preferences and handle the feelings that drive you to the refrigerator. These changes are far more valuable than quick, temporary weight loss. People who make sudden, radical changes in their diets will quickly burn out and regain a higher percentage of body fat than they had before they began. If you feel that you must force your self-control, pushing your logical will against your emotional desires, it is then only a matter of time before your defenses become fatigued and your emotions take over.

A sincere commitment to change the image you have of yourself, the quality of your life, and how you are motivated is far more important to achieving long-term weight loss and satisfaction with the lifestyle that keeps the weight off.

As an improvement over weight-loss diets, this chapter should serve as a guide to your individual efforts to gradually expand your food choices and preferences. In a 1990 study, Dr. Judith S. Stern, professor of nutrition and internal medicine at the University of California-Davis, found that the dieters most likely to keep off the extra pounds they had lost were those who had designed their own programs.

Expand Your Menu Choices And Decide on Food Values

Additions to your menu are most apt to become taste preferences when you add new foods gradually (one to two new items at a time) and become psychologically comfortable with them before introducing additional new food items. When you learn to *prefer* foods that help you, the mental struggle between what your emotions tell you that you want and what your logic tells you that you should eat is over. When you are at the grocery store, the cafe, or looking into your refrigerator and not using a structured diet, consider the following important factors in making decisions about what you want to achieve in your eating habits.

When you consider eating a new food (or any food), determine what is in it and what value it has for you. If you are uncertain of the contents or how it may affect your nutritional interests, don't buy it or eat it until you can find out. It may help to carry a small pocketbook on food values until you can make most of your decisions with ease. (But don't get caught up with number counting.)

When considering a new food or recipe, it is psychologically important to open your mind and free yourself of prejudgments and predeterminations. Telling yourself you won't like or can't stand a new food that will serve you well is a sure way to keep the old preferences. Remind yourself that you are adaptable! Your goal is to improve your belief that you can adjust your taste preferences to your physical and mental needs. Your self-talk and mental images can serve you in this effort.

Likewise, trying to convince yourself you love something new can also backfire. Allow for a neutral position by deciding you will repeatedly eat a new food for a six-to-10-week period before you make a judgment as to whether or not you like it. Give yourself time to accept it. Once you have accepted the food, continued use will lead to appreciation. Gradually, appreciation will become preference, as long as you are not talking yourself out of it. You have already come to like foods you once didn't. Use those memories to aid you. Let down your defenses — permit change.

Gradually Shift Evening Calories to Morning Hours

The time of day you eat is extremely important. The number and type of calories that can lead to weight gain in the afternoon or evening can actually help you achieve weight loss if you eat them during the morning hours. Your body needs more fuel and assimilates and burns foods better in the morning. Its efficiency wanes as the day wears on until you reach the danger zone of mid-afternoon to bedtime. Eating a larger, balanced breakfast and lunch is best achieved gradually. As you add to your morning meal, you are able to gradually alter your evening meal and the type of calories you consume at that time. Mental fatigue or tension at the end of the day adds to your appetite, so exercise or even a casual walk can reduce food drives.

Choose the Type of Calories
That Meet Your Needs

"Maintaining weight loss is the antithesis of counting every calorie," says Dr. Judith Rodin, chair of psychology at Yale University, as quoted by *American Health* magazine in the spring 1991 issue. All calories are not the same. Protein and complex carbohydrates burn two and a half times faster than fat. Complex carbohydrates are very difficult for your body to store as fat. They are stored as glycogen in the muscles and liver to provide energy that is quickly used. Also, one gram of fat has nine calories compared with four calories per gram of carbohydrate or protein. Protein must be broken down and reassembled before it can be stored, and this process burns calories. However, consider carefully your sources of protein. If you acquire your protein mostly from animal products, you will also get a great many unwanted fat calories, not to mention a lot of chemicals you don't need. The small amount of protein that you do need can be obtained from plant sources at a much lower cost in fat. Grains such as amaranth; beans such as defatted soy, pinto, and garbanzo; along with a few nuts, seeds, and sprouts will serve you well as sources of protein. Refined carbohydrates (sugars and flours) are empty calories you can do without; they, too, are easily stored as fat.

Prior to making your own healthful food choices, you may want to consider some of the findings from the unprecedented nutritional study in China.

Obesity is related more to *what* people eat than how much they eat. We're basically a vegetarian species and should be eating a wide variety of plant foods and minimizing our intake of animal products according to Dr. T. Colin Campbell of Cornell University. Dr. Campbell was the key U.S. figure in a cooperative epidemiological study with the Chinese and British. The preliminary findings are published in a book titled *Diet, Life-style, and Mortality in China: A Study of the Characteristics of 65 Chinese Counties*. This study looked at 367 factors in 6,500 Chinese subjects, dealing with lifestyle, nutritional intake, health status, and mortality since 1983. It is the biggest study of its kind ever undertaken and the results will be years in completion. The preliminary findings clearly point to the fact that the more animal fat we consume, the greater our chances of premature death from cancer, heart disease, and other major killers.

Allowing for height differences, the Chinese consume 20% more calories than Americans do, but Americans are 25% fatter. Americans eat more fat; Chinese eat more carbohydrates. The Chinese eat only 1/3 of the fat of the average American while eating nearly twice the carbohydrates.

In making your food choices, you might want to consider that the current recommendation by the American Dietetic Association that no more than 30% of calories come from fat may not be adequate for lowering the risk of heart disease and cancer. The China Study suggests a maximum of 20% of total calories from fat, but I'd recommend only 10% to 15% or less to minimize health risks.

A diet high in animal protein is linked to chronic disease. On the whole, Americans eat 1/3 more protein than the Chinese. It is the source of protein that makes the critical difference. Americans get 70% of their protein from animal sources, compared to only 7% for the Chinese. Based on this data, I'd recommend that we reduce our protein consumption, paying particular attention to animal sources.

Most Chinese consume no dairy products, obtaining most of their calcium from vegetables. They consume only half the calcium Americans do, yet osteoporosis is uncommon in China. Greater animal protein intake is associated with increased calcium needs. Dairy calcium intake does not reduce osteoporosis risk. In fact, it likely increases it. Vegetarians tend to have lower calcium needs and a lower risk of osteoporosis. High sodium intake also increases the need for calcium.

The range of blood cholesterol values in the U.S. population is said to be 155 to 274 mg/dL. Almost all the China group values are 88 to 165 mg/dL. Most importantly, according to Dr. Campbell, coronary heart disease risk in the China study continues to decline to an almost negligible level when cholesterol levels are low. Colon cancer risk correlates in exactly the same way. The study found less risk for disease in those who eat the least amount of animal protein.

Stay in Touch with Your Feelings and Knowledge

Understanding and sensing your nutritional needs leads to an ability to make sensible spontaneous choices in new situations. Understanding comes from collecting basic information and learning how to apply it to specific needs (e.g., you need carbohydrates to jog a 10K). You don't have to become a nutritionist; however, asking questions of one, reading a book or two on the subject, or taking a class will give you a good working knowledge. Once you have some general information, you can stay on top of new information by reading a monthly health magazine or a condensed nutrition newsletter. *Vegetarian Times, American Health,* and even the daily newspaper are good sources of current information. If you read what five different nutritionists have to say, you will find some differences and similarities. This can seem confusing, but remember, it is your unique body that really tells the story. Take into consideration all that you learn from the nutritionists, especially when you find most of them in agreement.

But even more important is listening to what your body tells you. Within twenty minutes to a half hour after you eat, your body will tell you how well it liked what you gave it. If you are becoming tense, tired, full of gas, etc., you know something disagreed with you. If your pulse is racing, you may be having an allergic reaction. The point is that nobody can know better than you how your food is affecting you if you learn to listen to what your body is telling you.

Think of Eating As an Adventure

Discovering how food works is much more exciting than the denial, forcing, controlling, and calorie counting that go with typical weight-loss diets. Your physical, emotional, and mental needs constantly change with age, levels of stress, pollution, physical activities, etc. Your adventure, then, becomes the search for the foods that will fuel your needs as they arise; always seek maximum performance, optimal energy levels, calmness, and health. As you are chewing on a carrot, imagine the brilliant orange color being tempered into a creamy sunshine sauce. Search for subtle qualities in foods that are good for you. Enjoy the juiciness of a nectarine and the snap of a piece of celery. You'll come to appreciate these healthful foods and even prefer them.

Using food to provide entertainment, companionship, emotional comfort, social rewards, sexual gratification, or to fulfill other non-nutritional needs leaves much to be desired. **As you make choices that meet your newly defined values, eating solely for nutritional needs provides its *own* joys and sensual satisfaction.** Moreover, you won't suffer frustration and guilt from expecting food to do what it cannot.

Devoting time and attention to what you eat is an important part of nurturing your self-esteem. You will build self-esteem by taking time to address your own food needs. You are worth the effort!

Rebel Against Your Old Self

Evolving your choices can help you create a more positive self-image. The system that works for you is not your controlling parents, spouse, boss, doctor, or the dietitian upon whom you may feel dependent. If you feel the need to rebel against something, let it be your old ways of thinking and behaving. You may not want to even be aware of such struggles going on because they may not seem to make sense to you. **If you join a weight-loss program because you feel too weak to help yourself, you are apt to come to both praise and resent that program and consciously or subconsciously rebel against it.**

Most of us don't want to be controlled. Perfectionists seek structure, which feels like control, because they don't trust themselves to perform well without a lot of guidelines. This way they can be sure to tell if they will get a gold star for their performance, that is, please others. If they start out doing well, then it is because of the program, but they are dependent on the program. Then they begin to resent the program on which they've become dependent because the dependency points out weakness in themselves. They become angry and fearful and rebel against the dependency and the controller (the program). Drop your defenses and allow yourself to see this is your *self-made* program.

Give Yourself Permission to Change

Allowing change in yourself works much better than forcing or controlling change. Forcing and controlling exhaust you and encourage your desire to stay with the old ways. To be in harmony of body and mind, thus achieving a relaxed balance of logic and emotion, let go of ego struggles and internal conflicts of right and wrong. Stop straining to avoid your fears. Move toward fears on your own terms. And don't force yourself to eat inappropriately (i.e., weight-loss diets).

CHAPTER 12

Guidelines for Healthful Food Choices

C hoose your foods for more than favorite tastes and
to satisfy your emotional needs. Choose foods for
lifelong healthful weight. In April 1991, Neal Barnard,
M.D., of the Physicians Committee for Responsible Medicine, proposed a new version of the four basic food
groups to prevent heart disease, stroke, diabetes, and
cancer. The proposed groups consist of grains, fruits,
vegetables, legumes, and no animal products. If you
learn only the following guide from which to select your
foods, you have enough information to make wise
choices. Simply keep a balance of the recommended and
recommended-in-moderation items from the various food
categories. And stay with quantities that meet your
body's needs, especially during the evening meal.

The foods listed below are divided into six major
categories: complex carbohydrates, proteins, fats and
oils, fiber, sweeteners, and liquids. Within the categories
are foods that are freely recommended, those that are
recommended in moderation, and those that you should
begin to "crowd out" of your diet. Remember, though,
that you must devise your own system of food choices
and that you will actually begin to crave healthy foods if
you practice without forcing yourself.

Consider several of the books listed in the bibliography if you want additional, more specific guidance for making food choices.

Freely recommended foods and beverages in the six categories below include fresh foods, free of pesticides when possible (though frozen foods can be fresher depending on storage and freezing methods); foods with high nutritional values and high fiber rather than calories from fat; and pure water (for drinking and cooking).

Foods recommended in moderation in the categories contain little or no refined carbohydrates, little or no refined sugars or flours, and little or no added salt or chemicals. Enjoy these foods occasionally, but make sure to monitor fat and toxin content. They may be higher than acceptable for frequent eating. In most cases, these would be avoided by a vegan vegetarian as well.

Foods that you should "crowd out" of your selections in the categories contain animal fat or refined sugars and are not recommended in a healthful diet; you may want to include them in the beginning, gradually eliminating them from your diet as healthful options increase. In the April 1991 issue of the *New England Journal of Medicine*, Dr. Walter Willett and Dr. Frank M. Sacks of Harvard University, from their research relating food to cancer and other illnesses, stated "the optimal intake of cholesterol is probably zero," meaning the avoidance of all animal products and fats — especially lard, red meat, and high-fat dairy products.

Complex carbohydrates should account for approximately 70% to 80% of your diet. Among the *recommended* complex carbohydrate choices are vegetables (especially greens), whole fruits, 100% whole grains, and legumes (e.g., peas and beans). Seeds and nuts will also provide complex carbohydrates, but you should eat these in *moderation*.

Recommended protein sources include defatted soy products like tofu, tempeh, and isolate; beans, peas, and lentils; 100% whole grains, such as rice, rye, millet, barley, amaranth, and quinoa; seeds and nuts like almonds and sesame; and sprouts, including vegetables, grains, and beans. In *moderation* you can also take protein from fresh fish (but not shellfish) and skim milk dairy products if you are not allergic. Protein sources that are *not recommended* and that you should gradually eliminate from your diet include cheese, which is high in fat and salt; no-fat cheeses, which are still hydrogenated and can raise LDL cholesterol; and meats, which contain a high percentage of fats and cholesterol and may also contain chemical preservatives, growth hormones, antibiotics, nitrates, and nitrites. Meat has a high association with major illnesses and causes calcium loss and other medical problems, such as certain cancers and cardiovascular problems.

For fats and oils, the less of these in your diet, the better. However, fruits are *recommended* for your needs in this category. Avocados are actually a fine source of oil, though they are high in fat. In *moderation*, choose cooking oils, preferably monounsaturated. A good choice is extra virgin, cold-pressed olive oil in a dark bottle, which helps avoid chemical breakdown from sunlight. Other sources of fats and oils taken in *moderation* include nuts and seeds, such as almonds, walnuts, and sesame; and whole grains. (Corn is especially high in oil though all whole grains have oil.) Fat and oil choices *not recommended* are all animal products, which are high in saturated fats, and saturated and polyunsaturated cooking oils.

The *recommended* sources of fiber are whole fruits, such as figs, prunes, and apples; whole grains, including oats, wheat, rye, and barley; vegetables like cabbage, broccoli, lettuce, carrots, and celery; and legumes including beans, chickpeas, and lentils. In *moderation*, enjoy nuts as a good source for fiber. But remember, they have a high fat content. Almonds and walnuts have the best nutrition. *Not recommended* are Brazil nuts, coconuts, macadamia nuts, and cashews.

As sweeteners, whole fruits are *recommended*, and you should eat as many as you like. Good choices are raisins, apples, and pears. *In moderation* you can turn to things like orange juice, honey, and maple syrup as sweeteners. But be careful with the last two. Even in their natural form they are high in calories that are easily stored as fat. *Not recommended* for sweeteners are sugars refined from grains, beets, sugar cane, and fruit as well as artificial sweeteners like aspartame (Nutrasweet) and sorbitol.

For *recommended* liquids, help yourself to as much water (up to 80 ounces a day) that you know is pure and clean, vegetable juices, caffeine-free herbal teas, and fat-free broths as you like. (Watch out for sodium in broth, though.) In *moderation* you can drink fruit juices and grain beverages like alcohol-free beer.

Quick Tips

Here are a few things to keep in mind when planning your healthful eating system:

- Grocery shopping is safer when you aren't stressed, fatigued, or hungry.
- Going grocery shopping once each week offers less exposure to temptation.
- Lean cupboards minimize tough decisions.
- Fattening foods, such as nuts, are better purchased in small amounts.
- When eating with friends, make your preferences known in advance.
- You will find when eating out that many restaurants will try to meet your needs if you give them a chance.

In the real world, of course, you can't always control the types of foods available to you or even where or when you can eat them. Your healthy eating system must also prepare you for making educated decisions when circumstances aren't determined by you.

Deciphering Labels

To make valuable use of the information on labels, you need some general information.

The U.S. Food and Drug Administration (FDA) is the primary regulator of food labels. Their original content came from the Federal Food Drug and Cosmetic Act of 1938. A major change in the layout and content of food labels was enacted in 1992.

Some major food items, such as meat and poultry, are not yet required to have labels at all unless they are part of a packaged or processed product; others, such as seafood, are usually not even inspected. Meat and poultry products are regulated by the U.S. Department of Agriculture (USDA). The Federal Trade Commission (FTC) regulates claims in food advertisements.

Marketers' overzealous efforts to appeal to shoppers looking for healthful packaged food and inadequate regulations or enforcement have often resulted in labels that are not only misleading and confusing but sometimes even fraudulent. Attention-getting words such as "no cholesterol" are emblazoned on packages of products that may actually raise your cholesterol level by being laden with other fats.

Nutrition labeling now appears on only 60% of processed foods. Even if a nutrition label has appeared on a package, it hasn't always been in a usable form. Labels have listed such things as grams of fat but provided no information regarding how much fat is too much.

Even if a label listed ingredients in descending order by weight, it often didn't tell the percentages that made up these rankings. Labeling practices such as these made it difficult for you to realize, for instance, that 50% to 75% of calories in ketchup is sugar or that mayonnaise is usually 100% fat. When foods, such as ketchup and mayonnaise have actually been improved by replacing vegetable oil, egg yolks, or sugar with more healthful ingredients, they can no longer legally use the names ketchup and mayonnaise.

Labels have often used misleading terms, such as "low" cholesterol, for which there was no legal definition. Labels didn't tell you that tropical oils, such as palm, palm kernel, coconut, and other saturated oils lead to fats in the blood. Cholesterol is found only in foods with animal products, but if you can't determine whether peanuts have been roasted in peanut, olive, or canola oil, you can only guess whether or not the nuts will have a cholesterol-raising oil in them. (Better yet, choose nuts that are not roasted or salted at all.)

Other terms, such as "high fiber," have also been misleading. One package may contain 1/10th the fiber of another brand of equal size and still have large red letters touting the fiber as though it were loaded with it. (Approximately 30 grams of fiber per day are recommended by some authorities.) Another confusing matter has been the amount of fat in products given as a ratio to the product's *weight*. What the consumer needs to know is the percentage of fat in the total *calories* of the product. For example, in "2% milk," 38% of total calories are derived from fat. If you are interested in limiting your fat to 20% or less of your total dietary intake, this kind of information is very important. Unfortunately, it has not been widely available.

On labels, the meaning of words such as "reduced," "light," and "natural" have also been confusing. With sodium, words like "very low sodium," "sodium-free," "salt-free," "no salt added," or "no salt" have not meant the product didn't contain sodium. The ingredients may have contained baking soda or soy sauce that could raise the sodium count significantly. Different forms of salt/sodium, such as monosodium glutamate, or MSG, are also found on labels in terms unfamiliar to the general public. The word "light" meant just about anything from more water to fewer calories, a paler color, a thinner cut, etc. A similar meaningless term has been "natural." In addition, the words "no sugar added" should never be taken at face value.

Another misleading promotion method has been indicating on the wrapper or the advertisement that the contents are "whole grain" or "real fruit." The whole grain or real fruit may be only a small percentage of the total volume. Although by weight it may have been listed first, it may have comprised only 4% of the calories in the product.

Manufacturers may use similar methods to confuse the consumer regarding oils. One example has been the phrase "may contain one or more of the following: olive and/or coconut and/or palm kernel oil." Olive oil has far less saturated fat than the other two, but you would have no way of knowing which oils were actually in the product and in what ratio.

"Natural flavorings" can mean just about anything. Natural and health food stores tend to sell products that can be trusted to a higher degree in terms of healthful qualities, but even here, terms like "natural flavorings" are commonly found, and adequate nutritional labeling has often been missing.

The nutritional labels themselves have often been hard to see or read because of the size of the print, where it is located, and the type of wrapper on the product. (It is difficult to read print on a transparent or shiny, bright, light-reflecting paper.) In addition, letters were sometimes run too close together, and often ambiguous wording was used without further explanation.

Sugar comes in many forms, and shoppers are confused when manufacturers list it by one of its many names: brown sugar; white sugar; honey; maple syrup; and grain syrups like rice and corn, barley malt, dextrose, sucrose, fructose. Whatever the type or name, it is still sugar and tends to have the same negative effects. It should also be noted that artificial sweeteners, such as sorbitol, aspartame (Nutrasweet), etc., have about the same calorie count as sugar by volume but a higher intensity of sweetness. As it relates to weight control, people who use artificial sweeteners tend to gain more weight than those who use regular sugar.

If a label doesn't give you the percentage of fat to calories in a product, the fat-finding formula for label reading begins by allocating 9 calories to each gram of fat. To calculate the percentage of fat calories, multiply the number of grams of fat by 9; divide by the total calories; then multiply by 100 to calculate the percent of calories derived from fat. It's really not even necessary to calculate beyond 9 calories for every gram of fat. Once you know that figure, just by looking at the total calories you can tell if the fat content is too high.

The new, federally required labels, which began implementation in the spring of 1993 and will be fully implemented by the spring of 1994, are focused on eating a healthy diet; old labels were concerned with vitamin deficiency. The new labels will only list vitamins A and C, calcium, and iron. It is mostly information about B vitamins that has been eliminated from the new labels. (Turn to green vegetables, whole grains, and beans to meet these needs.)

In place of the vitamin panel are guidelines for the consumption of the major health detractors in fat, cholesterol, sodium, and sugars, as well as contributors to good health like complex carbohydrates, fiber, and protein. These changes will enable you to eat wisely. Serving sizes will be standardized among similar products.

The Percents of a Daily Value section on the label shows how the food you select fits into your overall daily diet allowances. On the example label shown, if you consume 2,000 calories per day with a recommended intake of 65 grams of fat, the product provides 20% of the fat you are allowed for the day. Keep in mind, though, that the labels give a daily calorie guide as 2,000 calories, but men are generally recommended to consume 2,500 calories. Women should consume 1,900 to 2,200 calories each day. The guideline is also not suitable for children, the elderly, and athletes. Also keep in mind that you should limit the number of calories you get from fat to no more than 30%.

Treat each label as if it were a contract. Read the label carefully, do your calculations, and look for any tricks in the fine print. The point is, don't trust labels. Ask, learn, and eat fresh food whenever possible.

New labeling standards have done much to address past problems. They are now designed to be useful for the consumer, with standardized layout and even percentages of daily requirements for many nutritional ingredients including fat.

Nutrition Facts

Serving Size 1/2 Cup (114g)

Servings Per container 4

Amount Per Serving

Calories 260   Calories from Fat 120

	%Daily Value*
Total Fat 13g	20%
Saturated Fat 5g	25%
Cholesterol 30mg	10%
Sodium 660mg	28%
Total Carbohydrate 31g	11%
Sugars 5g	
Dietary Fiber 0g	0%
Protein 5g	

Vitamin A 4%   Vitamin C 2%   Calcium 15%   Iron 4%

*Percents (%) of a Daily Value are based on a 2,000 calorie diet. Your Daily Values may vary higher or lower depending on your calorie needs:

Nutrient		2,000 Calories	2,500 Calories
Total Fat	Less than	65g	80g
Sat Fat	Less than	20g	25g
Cholesterol	Less than	300mg	300mg
Sodium	Less than	2,400mg	2,400mg
Total Carbohydrate		300g	375g
Fiber		25g	30g

1g Fat = 9 calories
1g Carbohydrates = 4 calories
1g Protein = 4 calories

Grocery Shopping and Eating Out

When Louise dined out with friends and was asked, "Where would you like to eat?" in the past, she would usually answer, "Wherever you prefer would be fine with me." Always wanting to please others for fear of rejection, her answer had become a habit she did not think about.

Gradually Louise has become more assertive in taking care of herself and living closer to her own values. Now when she is asked, she discusses the matter and explains her interests and needs. Sometimes it will take a little longer to decide, or they may drive a little farther, but usually, at worst, a compromise restaurant will be picked. Often a friend will actually prefer a more healthful meal also. As far as I know, Louise has not lost one friend over her new assertive behavior, and she has discovered a few old friends are now easier to be with. She thinks more of herself for sticking more closely to her own values, and her healthful choices are becoming preferred. And she's losing weight. Louise's friends are also seeing her in a new light of greater respect, which frankly both surprises and pleases Louise.

Finding appropriate cafes has also been an adventure for Louise and her friends. At first, it was small changes, such as which pizza place had whole wheat crust and honored requests to go light on the cheese and top it with only vegetables. Then, it progressed to going where there was a salad bar with a really big variety and a fruit bar. The fresh seafood restaurants that would broil the fish were popular for a while, and, of course, the oriental cafes that would leave off the MSG and had a variety of vegetable dishes seemed like alternatives that most of her friends would go along with. Over time, however, Louise's choices have evolved into still more healthful choices. The meat, fat, sugar, and salt in most of her first choices became less acceptable. She learned about how polluted the fresh seafood from fish farms can be and how even cooking fish can create carcinogens. So she's decided to drop that alternative.

As Louise became more selective, the number of eateries in which she dined as well as the number of times she ate out declined; however, she did become more satisfied with the restaurants she did frequent. She knew what she wanted in each place and how to order when she would go to cafes that offered few choices that fit her new standards. Except for a couple of vegetarian restaurants, Louise used standard guidelines as she reviewed the menu offerings in new or less-than-desirable establishments. The first question was always, "May I get side orders that aren't on your menu?" The second question was, "Will your chef modify servings from your regular fare?"

One solution to the restaurant problem may be to go to a large chain grocery store. Many of these stores now have salad bars open at many hours of the day, or small amounts of produce and packaged goods or drinks may be purchased and taken back to the office or car to eat.

Larger food stores usually have a variety of drinks and packaged foods that are kept chilled. Such items as no-fat yogurts, fruit-flavored mineral water, whole grain muffins with raisins, etc., are available. Sometimes they even have tables in the store where you can eat. Walking through the grocery store to see how many new ideas or healthful foods you can find can be an adventure.

Many towns also have natural food cooperative stores. These, of course, are primarily food stores that are owned by the members who also often do much of the work of running the store and vote on the kinds of products the store will carry. These stores have been created not only to provide the most nutritious and clean food available (e.g., organic produce, etc.), but also to keep the cost of the food lower by joining with other co-ops to purchase in larger quantities. They are usually warm, friendly places that are often more relaxed than traditional supermarkets, and usually you will notice a friendliness with customers and clerks alike that will make you want to come back.

Health food stores, not to be confused with co-ops, are a mixed blessing to me. They often are the only place where certain health-oriented products can be found. I believe they serve a purpose and provide an alternative to the limited choices available in more traditional supermarkets. I also believe they have helped to bring about some long-overdue improvements by major food store chains in the products they sell and the contents of those products. The problem, though, lies with the consumer's tendency to accept the offerings without a critical eye.

Even in health food stores, you must read labels to know what constitutes healthful nutrition, especially according to your own definition. It is important not to count on the store clerk to diagnose or prescribe treatment for any symptoms or special needs you may have if this person does not have adequate credentials to do so. Do not seek magic from any product or jump to the conclusion that it is only the substances you ingest that are responsible for what ails you. Many factors influence your state of health and physical fitness. Easy, quick answers that seem too good to be true probably are — especially where weight problems are concerned. If you shop in health food stores, as I do, take the time to get to know the people who own and operate them. Know what you want and rely more on your own knowledge and that of your health-care practitioners (provided they are knowledgeable about nutrition). This is usually more reliable than information and opinions given to you by store clerks. I don't mean to condemn all health food store clerks or owners; some are very knowledgeable and may even have more training in nutrition than your M.D. However, practicing medicine is not why they are in business, and you need to be responsible for finding the foods that satisfy your personal needs. You need information from a variety of sources, and you must collect that information before making your decision about it.

Two less favorable options that I have felt compelled to choose at times are to have a small snack that I pick up at a health food store to tide me over until the next meal or simply to drink some clean water and miss a meal. If you want to lose weight, and the meal you skip is an evening meal, no physical harm should result. I do not recommend missing meals as a regular practice, and if you choose to fast for more than a meal or two, I recommend that you only do so under the supervision of a well qualified, experienced health-care professional — and never for the purpose of weight loss.

On the Road

Many of the same suggestions mentioned under "Eating Out" are even more appropriate in situations involving travel. Suggestions, such as requesting food choices not on the menu, dining in grocery stores, finding co-ops and health food restaurants, and even skipping a meal are all options that can be useful when you are on the road. More importantly, by developing options, you show yourself that you have choices. You feel better about yourself, which will foster even more sensible choices.

When I was a child taking trips with my parents, I remember my mother packing huge lunches that could have fed several children for several days. Usually all we would purchase would be beverages. My mother did this for economic reasons more than for health, but the idea has served me well on many trips.

Bringing your own food with you takes some planning and increases the amount you will have to carry, but it is being done more and more by all types of people who travel and are interested in healthful eating. Some celebrities will not only carry food for themselves and their families but will also bring cooking utensils and other equipment, such as blenders, to use in their hotel rooms. Many hotels provide kitchenettes for guests who want to prepare their own meals. In fact, many of the better hotels and motels have some rooms that come with a small refrigerator, sink, cupboards, and some type of small stove or microwave.

Grocery stores, health food stores, and co-ops are able to help you stock up either before you leave or when you arrive at your destination. When traveling by car, it is easier to take the perishable food already in your refrigerator, prepare hot-plate type dishes, such as vegetable stew, and eat in the car or the motel room. Coolers packed well with artificial ice can carry a great deal of food. Regular ice will also work, but it is messier and generally doesn't last as long.

Most of the time when you travel by airplane, flights are short enough that it is not necessary to eat during the flight. If, however, you are going to eat meals on the plane and you don't want to bring your own in your carry-on luggage, arrange to have special meals brought on board for you. You can do this when you purchase your ticket. Be forewarned that you may not always get the best, but usually it will be adequate. The airlines make a few too many different types of special meals. I have learned, for example, that just asking for a vegetarian meal does not assure me of healthful food. Either request that no fat or sugar items be included in your meal or inquire what will be served in their different special meal categories on your flight. You should be able to get something close to what you want. You pay handsomely for your in-flight meals. Most airlines have developed a system to conveniently handle your requests, so there is no reason to feel guilty about causing the airline to go to any additional trouble. Remember, the effort will make you feel better about yourself.

Whenever I arrive in a city or town on business or pleasure, I check the Yellow Pages under health foods and look for co-ops and health food cafes. If I do not find anything listed, I call a health food store close to where I am and ask if they know of any cafes, delis, or grocery stores where I might find the kinds of healthful foods I want. Usually there is at least one option reasonably close.

When visiting relatives and friends or dining out with them, it is certainly considerate to let them know about your food preferences and assure them that they need not go to any special trouble for you. If you stay at their home, do as you would at a hotel and bring as many of your special foods as is reasonable. Generally speaking, people who like you enjoy the opportunity to do something special to please you. I have also found that my friends and relatives like to know how and why I eat the way I do if for no other reason than they are curious. A little discussion about it is interesting to them as long as it doesn't turn into a lecture.

Dining out with business contacts or having a snack at the office during long meetings may pose more of a problem. In this situation, people still want to be helpful and even discuss it a little but much less so than in a social situation. This is when I have most often gone without a meal or snack. If possible, talking with the person who is providing or ordering the in-office lunch, rather than dealing with your business hosts, is your best chance to get what you want without putting anybody out or taking up pressured business time.

Special Occasions

Holidays, birthdays, and celebrations of every kind, unfortunately, often revolve around food and drink. We have a social tradition of believing that we are not having a treat, a "special" good time, or even tasty food unless we are "treating" ourselves to something unhealthy. Our attitudes and beliefs about what is "good" or "special" need changing as much or more than the food and drink we consume on these occasions. Weddings, promotions, graduations, babies, and even divorces and funerals are just some of these all-too-often special occasions. Any excuse to fall off the wagon can be found if one is really looking.

This is why it is important to learn to change food-choice preferences, not only on the basis of nutritional value but also on the basis of changes in taste preferences and changes in attitude.

When you truly believe you prefer the taste of healthful food, and you feel like you're having a treat when you're eating healthful food, then the struggle is over. You need no more advice, and you don't feel cheated or deprived.

Again, when possible, bringing your own food is good advice. Just be sure to let the hosts know ahead of time. Healthful, low-fat eating has become so commonplace that many hosts anticipate requests for it and provide something for their health-minded guests. Nevertheless, it is still wise to let them know ahead of time and offer to assist with some ideas at least. A food contribution would be even better. For potlucks, bringing a special dish that is both healthful and tasty will usually go over well. Non-healthful eaters generally get excited about healthful foods when they also find the food tasty, and usually they acknowledge their surprise and pleasure. Often they want to know where they can get this low-fat, healthful food or how to make it. If you choose your dish wisely, I am sure it will be a big hit.

Feeding Others

Entertaining people whom you know to be junk food junkies may be more difficult. I usually warn guests ahead of time and try to offer a wide variety of healthful items. If you provide a number of items, most people will be satisfied with enough of the food to enjoy the occasion. **It is very important not to change your own values and priorities. If you want to believe in yourself, it is important to live by your own values and accommodate others within those values.** I do not serve my friends and guests food or drink I know is unhealthy for me to consume. I will go out of my way to try to make it pleasurable and tasty, but I stick with the criteria that it must be healthful.

When I have asked clients in my office if they would knowingly serve health-damaging food to people they care about, the answer has generally been no. But, if we look closely at what they usually serve their guests on special occasions, the answer more accurately should have been yes. When asked that question, they assumed I meant something that would immediately make their guests ill. They didn't think about the slower killers such as fats, refined sugars and flours, alcohol, etc. Your guests may also enjoy the "new" healthful food because they see the occasion as a nutritional adventure. I have even had friends proudly boast later about the healthful meal they experienced, as though they had just eaten snake for the first time and had lived to tell about their enjoyment of it.

Without an adjustment to healthful eating as your *preference*, "occasions" stay special in part because of the unhealthful food. When healthful food becomes "special," "real food," the best-tasting food, and the food that is always preferred, it is only a matter of time before the "preferred" food is eaten most of the time.

No other person will ever be able to monitor your nutritional needs better than you. Louise has learned this. If you are ever to gain the confidence you want, it must come through your own insights and efforts. Therefore, it is important that you make the food choices necessary for your own well-being and not just to follow some authority's directives. If you need information, use professionals as resources, not as parental figures to be dependent on. *You* determine the choices and take responsibility to apply the information to your needs.

CHAPTER 13

Healthful Exercise — Loving It Your Way

While growing up, Louise was shy and non-assertive. Unless the teacher organized the playground games and required her to take part, Louise would retreat with a friend or keep to herself. She was working from junior high on, so she never took part in the usual extracurricular activities. Although she did have a bike, it was more for utilitarian purposes than for fun. Exercise was never something she enjoyed or at which she excelled. So is it surprising that as an adult she viewed it more like the physical work she did at home or on the job? Certainly exercise wasn't something she looked forward to or to which she wanted to devote her free time. This attitude was especially true when she became a postal worker where she spent most of her working day on her feet.

The more Louise learned about weight problems and the heavier she grew, the more she would try to *force* herself into a regular routine. In the various diets and programs she would join, her efforts would be short-term and often too rigorous. She would join fitness spas and aerobic dance classes, but soon the class time conflicted with other, higher priorities, or her friend wasn't able to make it, or something would interfere. Louise would then be disappointed in herself and put herself down for not being able to follow through with her commitment.

But after years of struggle with diet and exercise, Louise began to value exercise in a new way. Even when she was consistent for less than a few weeks, she knew her mood, energy level, attitudes, and hopefulness were noticeably improved. Her weight-loss efforts were clearly enhanced, her confidence level rose, and she found herself less often in those snacking kaffeeklatsches, cafes, or bars for entertainment. She knew how much more satisfying it was to identify with those people who value their health. Also, having read many articles and books, listened to testimonials and lectures, and counseled with exercise physiologists and weight-loss specialists, she believed that exercise was a worthwhile part of life. She was motivated and had given it a higher priority in her life. She even purchased a treadmill so that she would have no excuses about convenience, time, or appropriate clothing.

Louise injured her back at work while lifting a mail sack because her back had not been strengthened properly with healthful exercise. That is not to say that people who are in good physical shape can't be injured too, but usually injury happens less frequently. And when it does happen to more fit people, the injury is less serious and recovery more rapid.

After great medical expense, one operation, months of therapy, and pain that may never be completely gone, Louise is doing her exercises far more faithfully than ever before. Today she is happy just to be able to exercise at all. She is still deriving most of the benefits exercise provides and will probably continue to exercise as long as she is able — certainly not by forcing herself, which is not the recommended way to come to prefer exercise over being sedentary.

We realize, through experience, that body movement is the only way metabolism will be changed. Exercise is also part of the way in which we can find harmony in ourselves, and we come to love it. Dr. Judith S. Stern,

University of California-Davis, in studies from 1990, found the most important factor in permanent weight loss is physical exercise. Ninety percent of the people in the successful weight-loss group used regular exercise in keeping it off.

The psychology of exercise is getting your mind into the physical movements — not the payoff (e.g., being thin). We all have an athlete in us, and we discover it when we quit searching for it and find the joy in what is hard.

If I emotionally *want* to exercise, as opposed to simply thinking I *should* exercise, and I truly value exercise as a practical, important, and necessary part of my life and how I relate to others, there will be no question whether I will exercise. The questions will be only how it will fit into my schedule consistently and what are the best ways for me to do it. *Getting started* has everything to do with *staying with it.* Goals are more mental than physical. As with diet and weight loss, you are starting out to change the way you look at yourself, your beliefs, attitudes, and priorities, and not just your behavior or body shape. You are setting out to learn to *prefer* a new aspect to your life — to get beyond struggles with yourself. ("Will I or won't I exercise today?")

In every sense of the word, you are intending to get married to a behavior for life. You are wanting to become sensitive to your body and everything it can teach you. You want to learn how you and your body can nurture each other; you want to love, honor, cherish, and protect one another, through a lot less sickness and a lot more health, until death do you part.

This is a lot more and a lot better than simply forcing yourself through a routine you think you *have to do* until you lose weight. Forcing takes energy, it fatigues you, and it's only a matter of time until you quit. There are several components of your new approach to adding permanent exercise to your life.

Safety

Safety should be an overriding concern in your exercise program. **If you're injured, you can't continue to exercise, or at the least it disrupts the momentum of your program.** Additionally, if you exercise improperly, you not only expose yourself to injury, but the program won't work for you and you will burn out.

A logical starting place is to assess your physical fitness level and basic health. The only circumstances when it may be safe to forego a general physical exam and physical fitness check before starting any new exercise routine would be if you have a personal family physician you see at least twice each year and he or she gives you a green light with proper precautions, or if you are under 35 years old, have no personal or family history of cardiorespiratory, structural, or alignment problems; no physical symptoms; have been living a healthful lifestyle; and are no more than 20% above your ideal weight. Everyone, whether or not they fall into a group who may exempt themselves from a physical evaluation prior to starting an exercise program, should use caution and patience in seeking a good level of exercise. Remember, you have the rest of your life to do it. Also, if you do have a weakness that needs to be protected, seek guidance from an appropriate professional.

Decide on a Program

There are many options that will help you achieve a high level of health and fitness with good weight balance. Keep these considerations in mind.

- Do you have basic information about the activity?
- How convenient would it be for you?
- Is the cost within your budget?
- Will it provide you with balanced exercise?
- How much variety does it have?
- Can you do it anywhere?
- Can you do it alone?
- How much equipment is needed?
- Most of all, are you interested?

You may want to consider planning several different activities to meet your changing needs and to keep you from becoming bored or burning out. At the very least, it is advisable to make sure your exercise program is balanced. A good program will include stretching and limbering, aerobics, and contractual and firming activities. It will be progressive (can you do it more, longer, farther, etc., as your endurance builds?) up to the point where ideal weight is achieved. You may want to consider some activities for your training program that you can do any time or any place. Other physical activities, like team sports, could be social or entertainment experiences and done more occasionally. You wouldn't count on them to meet any of your physical or health needs; they would be for stimulation. Some very active people use their training activities to support their sports or entertainment interests. Training activities should not put you in competition with other people. It is *your* optimum you are seeking. You only want to win for you. Some activities you may want to include are:

- Walking/hiking/jogging/running.
- Biking/rowing/paddle boating.
- Stair climbing/jumping rope.
- Mountain climbing/skiing/skating.
- Swimming/water aerobics.
- Dance/aerobics (low-impact, with or without machines).
- Yoga/Tai Chi (a noncombative martial art).
- Weight lifting/circuit training.

All of these options are best done aerobically; most can be done either indoors or outdoors; all can be done alone; many can be done either with or without machines or other equipment; most can be done at either low cost or considerable expense; many are weight-bearing exercises, although some are primarily for the lower body.

Determine the Right Amount
Of Exercise for You

How much varies a great deal from person to person. A person who is generally in peak physical condition but is ill with the flu or other short-term illness should restrict exercise, as should someone who is in excellent general health but not physically fit. Your age, the time of day, whether or not you are rested, if you have any injuries, your level of knowledge of the skills or movements involved in the activity, your frame of mind or mood, how repetitive the activity is, and how much interest you have in the activity are also variables that might influence how much exercise is appropriate on any given occasion.

If you are in good health but just starting an exercise program, it is most important to not overdo it. In the first place, you are trying to learn the movements correctly so that you don't end up stiff and feeling unable to perform the next session. Going slowly while you determine your optimal starting point gives you time to make psychological adjustments. It is more important to want to repeat the exercise than to see how much you are able to do or how fast. Try starting at three exercise sessions each week and building to five or six days each week while you are trying to lose weight, taking extra days off from time-to-time after you have achieved your weight goal. How much exercise you do during each session should also be progressive at an appropriate speed until you reach your ideal weight.

It doesn't matter how little time you spend on your exercise routine to start with. Even five minutes is fine, as long as you add minutes each time you are able to do your routine easily. Work up to at least thirty minutes per session. For peak condition, work up to one hour. Distance and speed are variables of "how much" and can clearly affect the duration and difficulty.

For the person losing weight, inappropriate speed, distance, and level of difficulty could bring greater possibilities of injury or psychological burnout. *Gradual* is the key and progressive and consistent the goals. You can be a star tomorrow. Be a person who learns to love exercise first.

Decide on the Best Time to Do It

When to do it includes some interesting options. Those who are most consistent with their routine tend to exercise in the morning. Morning exercisers are up to 75% more consistent than those choosing to exercise in the late afternoon or evening. On the other hand, those who exercise in the morning are more prone to injury. By afternoon or evening your connective tissue will be warmed and less tight, though with age, connective tissue warms more slowly.

It is even more important to be flexible with your routines. To become rigid or compulsive about when you do your exercise sets you up for stress, disappointment, and excuses for not doing your routine or burning out fast. This is why counting on set class times, counting on a friend, or counting on ideal weather tends not to work. Always have options so you don't have to forego your exercise if one or more factors aren't favorable. Vacation time, business trips, or having guests in your home can also be excuses to procrastinate or quit. Routines are better kept throughout the year, no matter what the circumstance (except illness). **It is very important to your own self-worth to see yourself make time available to do your routines, especially if you are stressed and short of time. This is the only way you convince yourself of the importance of exercise and the fact that you are worth the trouble.**

Seasons can also dictate a change in the time of day you choose to exercise. The number of hours of daylight, the hours you work, and the type of exercise you choose all have an effect on when you do your exercise. Be Flexible! Be Consistent — Not Rigid! Fit exercise into your schedule when you can, but fit it in. Barring illness, missing more than twice a month can indicate you are having to push yourself to do it and are not giving it a true priority. Let exercise be in your life!

Select a Place to Exercise

Where to exercise includes many choices in the short term, but there is really only one choice for the long term.

In the nineties, the world is more geared to exercise than ever before. We have commercial fitness centers, parks and recreation programs, private athletic clubs, tennis and swim clubs, community centers, school fitness centers and tracks, PAR courses, aerobic dance classes, hotel and airport workout rooms, corporate exercise programs, biking-walking-jogging-hiking-cross-country-skiing clubs, rowing teams, water aerobic classes, neighborhood walking groups, hospital health promotion programs, athletic medicine clinics — all wanting you to get in shape.

These are wonderful facilities and organizations, but they all have limitations, which means you are not likely to stay with them for the rest of your life. Many of them cost money, they are available only at certain hours, they have lines of people, they have good and bad instructors, they can become more of a social than a physical exercise, they go in and out of business, what you can do there is often limited, machines may be broken or overcrowded, you're expected to keep pace with the others, and the list goes on. None of them are as right for you as the place where you are.

If you are going to exercise for life, you need to be able to do it at work, on the road, and, especially, at home — the one place you are most apt to stay with it. All those other places are all right to use for variety and special needs, but don't count on them or come to feel you need them.

Choose Whom to Exercise With

There are not as many choices to make in terms of choosing exercise companions. Public or commercial places put you together with strangers, and that may or may not be a good motivator for you. Your friends and relatives may or may not be available to exercise with you. Sooner or later the timing will be off. Some people may be able to afford a personal instructor or motivator. Some people follow TV instructors. Some buy videos to use at home. Some have teachers at school or in the fitness centers. **But the only one you can count on being there for sure is the one in the mirror.**

Using well-qualified instructors for a while to get you started is a wise idea. Instructors in books cannot see you and often leave out important individualized information. Friends, spouse, kids, dogs, and neighbors are unlikely to have enough training to give you good information and will only motivate you in the short term, at best. If you have these people with you for a while, enjoy them and get the most out of them. In the long run, though, plan to be your own main person in your own lifelong program — your own friend, teacher, and above all, motivator. I know people who have been waiting for years for their friend or spouse to exercise so they can get started. This is your life and nobody else's.

Choose a Source of Information

Among your sources of information are books, magazines, videos, exercise facilities, equipment manufacturers, and exercise specialists. Don't let your guide be your buddy who has been exercising two weeks longer than you. The wrong advice could lead to injury, ineffective development, hard-to-break habits, a dislike for exercise, or quick burnout. I encourage you to read a book on the subject before you choose either an instructor or facility. Make sure the book, like the instructor or facility you choose, has excellent credentials. Criteria should include information that has been well researched, recognition from known authorities in the field, academic credentials, ample, appropriate experience, and testimony by satisfied students or clients. If you read up on the activity you want to incorporate into your program, you will require less time with an instructor, you will learn faster, your questions will be fewer and more pertinent, and your expectations more realistic. Having a personal or classroom instructor provides you with someone who can observe you, guide you, correct you, and help you to reach your potential. If your instructor works where you practice, you will have ongoing attention and someone to help monitor your progress. Remember, just because an instructor is well qualified in one activity, it does not mean he or she is an expert in all exercise activities. Specialists can save you time, frustration, money, and possibly injury.

The best all-around help I have been able to find in my community has been at the fitness center at my local community college. The instructors are highly trained in a variety of activities. They are there every day and have access to resources that supplement their personal skills. They protect me in every possible way, they help one another, and we develop a personal working relationship. And all this comes at a very low cost compared with the alternatives.

Select the Proper Clothing and Shoes

Clothing and shoes are not always necessary when you are exercising in the privacy of your home. Exercising in the nude can be a wonderful, freeing experience if you have comfortable rugs or mats and you either live alone or have a partner who appreciates the fun or values the non-conformity of it. The views and poses are unusual, and if you try it once, you may want to do it again. This is certainly not a requirement, or for everybody, but remember, changing you means not only establishing exercise routines but also changing some of the attitudes that may have held you back.

If you plan to exercise outdoors and in public places, the right clothes and shoes will not only provide modesty but also protect you from the elements and foot damage. Clothes can also help you look good, which is part of the reason most people exercise in the first place. Practical, colorful, attractive clothing and shoes can also stimulate you simply because you know you look good and color enlivens us. If, however, your main concern with clothing is for social reasons or to look sexy, your motivation may benefit from some reexamination.

Bright, luminescent colors are practical at night when jogging or riding a bike on the side of the road. Tight fitting materials can keep you from getting hung up in equipment or causing other accidents, yet they provide excellent freedom of movement. Gortex and other relatively new materials do an excellent job of keeping your muscles warm without overheating, removing the excess water from your skin, and promoting evaporation. This will protect against such things as hypothermia in cool weather and chafing in warm weather. Your body burns calories to keep a stable temperature in cold weather and flushes water in warm weather. Avoid over-dressing in either type of weather just to cover up un-wanted pounds.

Nothing is more important to lifelong exercise than your feet, knees, and legs. If you have the right footwear for the right activity, it can go a long way to-ward keeping you injury free, helping you enjoy your workouts, and reaching your optimal performance levels. This is especially true for the overweight person. The right fit for width and length, along with sufficient sup-port to keep your foot stable but flexible, with ample cushioning to absorb the pounding is a tall order. Unfor-tunately, all of these requirements in a single shoe that has good durability can be costly, especially when some recommend that new shoes be purchased every three months or 200 miles, whichever comes first. With prices ranging from $30 to $150 and more per pair, look for a discount store that carries your brand.

Wearing worn out or inadequate footwear could, on the other hand, lead to expensive medical bills and con-siderable pain. So seek out the best personal guidance possible to make sure you select the right footwear for the right sport. Some possible sources of guidance are podiatrists, training books and manuals, specialty maga-zines, or organization newsletters. Some stores that spe-cialize in carrying a wide selection of footwear for all popular exercise activities in a good range of prices have at least one sales clerk who has a fundamental knowledge of the shoes. But this person won't know your feet, knees, and legs. If you have special problems with these areas, I strongly suggest you see a podiatrist or orthopedic or athletic medical doctor who exercises regularly. Special gear such as orthotics (foot supports) should be specially made for your feet.

Waist belts, wrist supports for joint protection, and headbands to keep the sweat out of your eyes can help too.

Choose the Right Equipment

Equipment is essential to any well-balanced personal exercise and fitness program. As I stated before, fitness is not just weight loss; it is *fat* loss. Firming, shaping, and aerobic exercise, along with stretching and limbering are all necessary. It is important to be able to exercise where and when you want. Instead of being able to find convenient excuses *not to* exercise, give yourself convenient excuses *to* exercise.

It is not my intent to discourage the use of or membership in a public or private fitness center. I am a member of one myself. In addition to the training, I enjoy the social aspects of working out with other like-minded people and even use it as a place to discuss business. Also, I could never afford, nor do I have space for, all that beautiful, chrome-plated equipment. However, if you restrict yourself to a certain place, specific hours, or requiring the presence of other people, your chances of continuing to exercise on a regular basis are greatly reduced. These restrictions are also a statement about your commitment.

When you are without special exercise equipment, workouts can also be done by using your body as a weight, walking, jogging, or improvising with chairs, suitcases, door frames, and such. But it is much harder to get a full, balanced workout, and psychologically, it is not nearly as motivating as being able to do your own routine with ease. The longer you exercise, the more refined your skills, knowledge, and sensitivities become. You know when you've had a good session and how to get at those places that need more work. So your appreciation of good, versatile, durable equipment grows along with your physical development.

Because weight loss is personal, there are many reasons why your best chance of keeping those extra pounds off is through setting up your own program. Being able to exercise on your own is a key aspect of your main goals of fitness and health. There are many optional pieces of equipment that can give you a workout at home, but most of them have drawbacks, such as the price, size, and portability.

About ten years ago, I was traveling a great deal in my work, and it seemed as though I just could not get to the fitness spa I was using at the time. I wasn't home to use my own equipment, and most of the portable equipment I tried to take with me was far too limited. What I found on the road was very hit-or-miss, and usually with my schedule, I just wasn't getting my exercise routine in. Then one day I discovered a wonderful little two-pound bag of exercise equipment that would provide me with the means to achieve all the benefits of exercise I could expect to find in a complete fitness center.

Its inventor, Bobby Hinds, called his creation the Lifeline Gym™. It was an ingenious arrangement of rubber ropes that could be easily configured into resistance training equipment. The Lifeline Gym™ is portable, weighing only two pounds, and disassembles into a small carrying case you could hold on one finger for hours and could travel with anywhere. It is adaptable to almost any environment, any type of exercise movement, or any person. It could work in a hotel room, office, home, even on a camping trip — anywhere with ten square feet of space.

I can make any exercise movement that I do at the spa, have heavy or light amounts of resistance, and change exercise rapidly to speed up the amount of time I spend doing it. There are no heavy weights to do damage to me or property. It's extremely durable, with no mechanical parts to break down. The cost is very low;

the equipment requires little or no storage space and can be put out of sight easily.

Probably the part I liked best is that it can provide an aerobic workout, as well as muscle development, toning, and shaping. It comes with what is described as a "treadmill belt," only it is like no treadmill I have ever seen. It allows the user to move around from side-to-side or walk or run backward or forward. It doesn't require that I hold on to bars to avoid falling down, and it even gives me the freedom to answer the phone or change channels on TV without skipping a step.

It is so simple, so adaptable to individual needs that anybody can use it — from a little elderly lady to the most powerful professional athlete. It can even be used in rehabilitation from injuries. Knowledgeable exercise physiologists think it is great, too, for it meets special needs for proper training, such as full range of motion, resistance, and quick adjustment from zero to hundreds of pounds. It also comes with a complete exercise guide book and wall chart, so the user knows what he or she is doing and why and how to do it correctly. Finally, it leaves no room for excuses for not exercising, barring illness.

When you can do your exercise privately, you need not impress anyone with how much you can do, how you look, or if you have the latest clothes. When I injured my knee and couldn't run, I could still lift my legs a half inch off the carpet, move them a very short distance, and manage to get an excellent aerobic workout with the Lifeline Gym™.

Years later this product is still on the market and still at a very low price; only now it is even better. The equipment is made out of better materials and it is even easier and safer to use. Yet my old one is not worn at all, is easy to use, and I've never come close to hurting myself with it. In addition to everything else, it now comes with a video showing how to use it, a 20-minute body-building routine, and a 20-minute aerobic workout done by experts in the field.

For the person serious about getting the weight off for good and taking up exercise for life, I know of no better equipment at anywhere near the price. The best way to get a Lifeline Gym™ is to call toll free to 1-800-553-6633. Tell them your age, size, and your needs, and they'll mail you a gym that is just right for you. If you prefer to write, mail your request to:

Lifeline International, Inc.
1421 South Park Street
Madison, Wisconsin 53715

Establish Harmony Between Mind and Body

Body/mind harmony is essential to the lifelong enjoyment of exercise as an integral part of your lifestyle. To have harmony between your mind and body is to be balanced and calm, with your energy focused. When the process of movement is the inner joy, and not just the pride and ego satisfaction after it is over, no question exists whether you will or won't exercise.

Adding exercise permanently to your life usually means something else may have to be reduced, changed, or eliminated. If you let go of some self-defeating activities in favor of exercise, you have an even better chance that your restructured priorities will last. If, like Louise for example, you let go of Friday evening out with friends (a fattening supper and a few drinks at the bar), you may miss the old times for a while until you make new friends at the fitness center and start getting in shape. When you rejoin your old friends a couple times, you will most likely find that your progress and pride in your personal changes are likely to result in less need to return to "Friday night out." As you establish friendships with new people who share a common interest in healthful living, some of your old friends may drift out of your life. Others may join you at the fitness center. Changing one aspect of your life will, in some way, affect other aspects of your life. At first it does make it hard, but because it is hard, when you are successful in making a change, you will be more impressed with the changes you've made and your self-esteem will raise even higher.

Measure Your Progress

Progress and the factors that influence it are easily observed by you and others. Unfortunately, the one thing that most weight losers go by is the bathroom scale. **If you are interested in long-term success and finding what your capabilities really are, a scale will be the least of your concerns.** Your clothes and a mirror will tell you if you are the weight you want to be. What you see and how you feel tell you much more than a scale or tape measure.

More difficult to observe, yet far more important, is what goes on underneath the skin and in your mind. What you really want to lose is *fat*, not just weight. Fat loss can't be measured by a scale, tape measure, or visual observation. Weight loss without exercise can easily lead to a higher percentage of your remaining body weight being composed of fat as opposed to muscle and water. Without exercise, even bone density can become less. If you squeeze someone who has an average height-to-weight ratio but has done little or no exercise, they could feel like mush. Muscle is denser and heavier than fat. It is made up mostly of water and protein. Protein and the carbohydrates that fuel muscle burn two and a half times as fast as fat. So, if you are not exercising while losing meaningful amounts of weight, the muscle loss will be much greater than you want.

There are several good methods for assessing how much of your weight loss is fat. One is a body composition analyzer, which is an electronic instrument that works much like sonar in ships. Input your correct gender, weight, height, and age, and in a few seconds it can give you an assessment of your weight broken down into water, muscle, and fat percentages. Weight-loss facilities and fitness centers now commonly have either the body composition analyzer or hand-held calipers to measure percent of body fat. Calipers work like the pinch test with your fingers, measuring the fat in a one-inch pinch at key sites on the body. A mathematical formula can give you a fairly close measurement. Probably the most accurate means of measuring body fat, if done correctly, is water weighing, usually done only at a hospital, university, or sports medicine facility. It is more expensive, takes much longer, and has the added inconvenience of having you don a bathing suit, hold your breath, and be dunked under water for longer than most people like.

You should also remember that exercise may bring enough muscle gain while you are burning fat that weight loss seems slower than you would expect at times. A tape measure can usually alleviate concern if your measurements improve even though your weight goes up or stays the same.

Other measurements of your exercise progress are more subjective. They include things like increased energy level, your endurance on hard days, your sense of well-being, your attitudes, how you handle stress and depression, your sexual appetite, coloring, humor, and, with some people, possibly even your resistance to colds and flu. Other factors are more important to long-term success. They include your growing appreciation for your exercise routine as seen in your attitudes about doing it, the priority exercise takes when you're pressed for time, how you talk to other people about it, and how much you seek new challenges in your exercise program. Most important of all for long-term success is how consistently you look forward to doing it, miss it when you don't do it, and whether you turn to exercise or food when you are distressed.

How well you progress in your physical development, the appreciation you hold for exercise, and how long you continue it are important factors that can be influenced by many things, some of which you may not have considered.

- Approval and support from important people in your life.
- Your nutritional habits.
- Work habits and requirements.

- Travel and adjustments for it.
- Social and religious involvements and adjustments.
- Involvement and modeling attitudes within your family.
- Where you live (climate and community) and on and on and on.

Progress can be slower or faster, easier or harder, depending on these variables.

As with dieting, *gradual* is the operative word in change. Your body changes are gradual so you don't injure yourself, get stiff and uncomfortable, or suffer psychological burnout. Gradual change also gives you time to make mental adjustments that allow you to find the joy in your changes.

Many Roads Lead to Mastery

The approaches to developing a true commitment to exercise are many and varied. Following are just a few examples.

- Frequently adding variety in time, place, and activity helps. The same basic movements can be done in many ways.
- Exercise with a partner, group, or alone.
- Keep expectations for yourself minimal. Make decisions about your progress as you go.
- Avoid comparisons or competition. It only leads to burnout and emotional stress.
- Learn to focus on what is happening within yourself; be sensitive to your physical or emotional self.
- Fantasize and imagine the now, and envision the path you want to walk.
- Involve yourself with your environment, for example, air, birds, sounds, terrain.
- Practice meditation or self-hypnosis (apart from or during exercise).
- Let go of mental conflicts (struggling with yourself about whether or not you will exercise today or not).

- Value the process more than the outcome.
- Strive for mastery, taking a regular practice and turning it into a discipline, helping yourself to let go of your need for instant gratification.

All the above suggestions may help you to incorporate exercise in your lifestyle, but probably none is as important as the last — mastery.

This idea certainly applies beautifully to the role of exercise in effective weight-change efforts, but once the concept is understood, it is easy to see how it applies to all other aspects of self-change.

Dr. George Leonard is the person responsible for bringing this profound concept to my attention in his book entitled *Mastery*.

In Dr. Leonard's view of mastery, several aspects are most relevant to developing an intrinsic change.

- Let go of our addiction to the quick fix and our never-ending, never-fulfilling quest for a series of climactic moments.
- Find a natural rhythm or harmony of life instead of attempting to force, control, or contain behavior.
- Return again and again to a discipline or task, even when we appear to be going nowhere.
- Live more fully in the present moment with keener awareness and sensitivity to our world.
- Become aware that learning is going up and down. There will be a little less down after each new, higher up, and we will spend a lot of time on plateaus with some climaxes along the way, with no real end, just continual growth and learning.
- Practice in a centered, balanced way — unrushed — focused on the movements, not the outcome. Know the path on which you walk.
- Make a connection between the practice of mastery and positive social transformation. Focus on the moment and greater awareness will result.

Dr. Leonard uses the martial art discipline of aikido as a base for transformation, but anything from gardening to meditation to stamp collecting to art will do. And, of course, mastery certainly applies to exercise. It is something you do on a regular basis, not casually, but not competitively either. The mastery is really within you, a path that leads you toward knowing yourself.

My years of morning yoga, aerobics, and weight lifting truly let me know who I am, just as Louise is learning to know herself, and just as you can learn to know yourself. We are all in a constant, unending state of becoming. We will always be able to find something new and more stimulating from the routines of what we do. Choose something and do it, and do it, and do it, without expecting anything more than what you get from doing it over and over, and the rewards will come.

CHAPTER 14

The Answers?
From Control to Harmony

What Ever Happened to Louise?

L ouise is changing. She is changing her life and her habits, and she has stopped struggling with herself, with her husband, and with her work. Louise, the consummate perfectionist, no longer needs to control and manipulate her way through life.

Eating for health is now an adventure, and her newly developing capacities in aerobic exercise excite her. Louise is starting to focus on her own intrinsic motivations for day-to-day decisions. Most important of all, she trusts herself more with each new day. She has been living up to her own values because she sees herself go through long periods staying true to her practice when it is hard, inconvenient, and especially when she feels she is making little or no progress. She knows, now, that she can count on Louise, which makes it much easier to face her fears, especially the fear of possibly failing.

Part of her solution is that Louise has allowed herself to become involved with a discipline in a way very different from compliance to weight-loss diets and exercise routines. With mastery of a discipline, in her case Tai Chi, she is not after any greater goal than the joy of the movement and the satisfaction of practicing the process. It isn't a matter of control and forcing herself through each practice to achieve praise; she practices because she wants to — even when her improvements are very slow. Breakthroughs occur when they are not expected, and Louise has become more skilled, *but that isn't the point.*

Something else is happening. The longer Louise practices, the more she finds a *calmness* that was never there when she struggled to meet the expectations of a weight-loss effort. She has also become more sensitive to her own feelings and has found changes in most other areas of her life. She is starting to believe in herself and the fact that achieving her goals comes as a by-product of her efforts along the way.

Problems with eating, exercise, relationships, sex, etc., are still there but not to the degree they once were. Fears still come up, and she doesn't like them any better, but the way she deals with them is more effective. She does not react to them by overeating. Louise has turned her focus inward and balanced it with her outward focus. She no longer doubts herself. She knows she will sometimes make mistakes, and she also knows she will recover from them. *Control* is no longer necessary.

Louise is not fully where she wants to be yet and is happy to know she may never be. But her impatient struggle has stopped.

Another benefit of these changes is that Louise has lost 40 pounds and kept them off for four years. She would like to lose five more pounds, but she is no longer after the instant gratification of quick weight loss. Louise has no doubts about the rest coming off or that she will be able to keep it off. Conquering her weight is no longer a struggle. Louise is learning she will be whatever she wants to be.

Earl, Louise's husband, has more than noticed the changes — not just in her weight, but in the way she uses her time, the comfortable attitude she has about people, and her confidence in herself. Earl knows he has some decisions to make about himself now. Louise has moved mentally and behaviorally to a different, healthier place. Does he want to move on, too, or continue to be separated from her and her life? He is coming to realize that it is really what he wants for himself that is important. If he gets to a better place with his own life, it can only improve his relationship with Louise. What he hasn't considered yet is that no person stands still in life; he either grows and changes or he moves backward. Both forward and backward are risky, but forward has hope.

Louise has a momentum going now. She has an energy and a belief in herself that is building and can carry her through each new problem and fear. Her back may never be perfect and her work may be filled with peaks and valleys, but she has learned she has the magic inside herself to carry her along with a quality to her life that makes it worth living.

Weight Loss through Wellness

The weight loss through wellness method can be categorized in many ways, and no matter how the many aspects of it are organized, there is no set order that is right for everyone. This is especially true because needs keep changing, and only the person who experiences the needs has the potential to be aware of what is needed at any given moment. Ownership of wellness cannot be given away. Therefore, you must complete the steps outlined below to self-change and growth in the order and speed that best suit your needs. You could work on several at once, or you could work on one at a time.

Before starting on any one aspect of each of the steps, it may be useful to pick out those areas that are in the most or least urgent need of attention as a way of getting started. The steps start and end with your philosophy of life. Your persistence and determination in completing all eight steps will earn you the belief in yourself. As in all cases of self-change, *you are the boss*.

You may need to seek still greater detail from other local resources to understand and bring about these changes. Your initiative in finding information and taking action as you feel a need for it is a crucial factor in bringing about the change you seek.

- SELF-AWARENESS: In the *long term*, self-awareness deals with the underlying causes that can make you vulnerable to becoming more easily stressed, more strongly stressed, and having stress last longer. Ongoing causes are a need for belief clarification, value-priority rankings, decisions to achieve self-esteem, and understanding the whole person and existential self.

  In the *short term*, self-awareness has to do with the minute-to-minute situations of each day and how you generate or handle your emotions based on what you experience and your perceived ability to cope with those perceptions. These factors are monitoring self-talk, monitoring mental pictures, monitoring emotions, and cognitive modification of perfectionistic behaviors and thinking.

- HEALTH, FITNESS, AND NUTRITION: The obviousness of these factors does not diminish their power and importance. Learn healthful eating and exercise. Develop a sensitivity to your body's needs. Develop healthful taste and exercise preferences gradually. And achieve medical self-care education and treatment ownership.

- EMOTIONAL OWNERSHIP: Practice daily stress reduction techniques. Be aware of your control over your behavior. Build a support system.

- COMMUNICATION SKILLS: Practice being open, honest, and tactful in expressing feelings. Learn to clarify your thoughts. Practice assertiveness and be aware of what you're communicating with your body language.

- SELF-IMAGE BUILDING: Acknowledge and identify your own fears. Desensitize those fears by taking small risks, such as social adventures. Explore what has meaning or purpose or leads to a feeling of aliveness.

- PEAK EXPERIENCES: Be open to peak experiences in all realms of your life: physical, intellectual, social, psychological, and spiritual. Don't overlook playfulness and humor.
- OWNERSHIP OF PERSONAL FREEDOM (Existential Reality): You exercise personal freedom by making choices and decisions, your commitments, taking responsibility for your actions, self-improvement, getting outside yourself, and by just experiencing life.

Meaning comes from what you give to life, what you take from life, and the stand that you take toward your condition.

The wellness lifestyle can include many aspects of well-being, which can be broken into many categories. It can be customized to suit your life, values, and beliefs, which means it can be developed to work for you.

Wellness is more than an academic or intellectual approach based simply on the accumulation and application of appropriate information. It is empowerment because it gives you the power to make life choices. The loss of weight or maintaining healthful weight balance need not be the intended purpose of achieving a wellness lifestyle. Those aims will be realized as a natural by-product of living the wellness lifestyle.

With mastery, the focus is on the practice of the discipline. In empowerment, the focus is on the understanding, development, and practice of a self-enhancing attitude. The focus of this method is health. How healthy can you be? On one side of a health continuum, humans may fall into levels of illness with anything from a hangnail to premature death. At the center we have the absence of illness — a body without disease, mind and body parts that are not malfunctioning in any observable way, a neutral point. But beyond this are levels of wellness. For a great many people this is an area that is totally unexplored. Don't let this be true of you.

Doing It on Your Own

Doing it on your own is just that — doing it alone. It is never really possible to avoid making your own decisions and owning responsibility for them if you want to take credit for the outcomes. This does not mean you can never learn from others or listen to their opinions. Can you solicit support? Yes, in the same way you talk about your day when you come home in the evening. All kinds of resources can be brought into this process. But without the risk of self-initiated action to experience what you believe you understand, you will have no emotional integration in your beliefs about yourself. In other words, you would continue to perceive yourself as you have, with self-doubt and low self-esteem.

Control or Harmony?

Most commonly encountered methods, techniques, or practices to bring about change in emotions, behavior, or self-concept tend to be (magic) from others that will require no risk taking and no confronting of all the frightening possibilities. At the same time, by even seeking magic, we reinforce feelings of self-doubt and reduce self-esteem. We are concluding that we are incapable of changing ourselves. How to handle this difficult, frightening dilemma and what Louise has been doing through her mastery are what this chapter is about.

Ironically, in some ways, we are seeking that which we already are — nothing more than being ourselves. I mean truly being who we are without any covers, pretenses, or fears of not meeting the expectations we think others have for us. It seems too risky in a competitive "winner-versus-loser" world to live by our own beliefs, values, and intuitive decisions after a lifetime of being rewarded for pleasing others and trying to make ourselves lovable instead of learning how to love.

Leaping that chasm where we disconnect from the familiar and hurtle through unknown space is often seen as too risky. We're trying to find an orientation to begin anew without dropping into the abyss or smashing into

a rock wall but touching down gently to make a successful beginning on the other side.

This change, a risky leap, can be helped by insights
and understanding — maybe even some practice. The
decisions, the action, the ending of what you were hanging on to that kept you overweight and frightened must
be your own. Confronting the fear of reorienting and
starting anew must be your own. If you do not experience yourself going through this process, you will have
no emotional integration of what you have come to understand intellectually. In an attempt to avoid risk, fearful people seek control through structured, organized
diets and programs. These almost always backfire.

Control, as I've mentioned, does not seem to be effective in the long-term for bringing about change. The
small percentage of those who bring about long-term
change by controlling themselves and their environment
experience a great deal of ongoing stress and inner conflict. Some proponents of control methods have a saying
that sums up the problem very well: "Live one day at a
time." Whether controlling is an external or strictly internal struggle, the results seem to be about the same.

**There is a difference between control and har-
mony. It is like the difference between dancing to
music by envisioning the foot marks on the floor and
counting the steps with the beat versus moving to
the rhythm of the music as you feel it without the
fear of taking a wrong step.**

In Louise's case, she went from trying to have others
control her (which didn't work) to trying to structure and
control herself (which didn't work) to finding a *harmony*
through a discipline (which did work). How and why did
this happen? Wasn't she still receiving assistance?

An old country western song has a line that seems
to answer the question: "I long for the freedom of my
chains." In other words, once *she* chose a direction for
herself and gave it a purpose and meaning, she was no
longer just a leaf blowing in the wind. Each new weight-
loss program or product had lasted until a stronger wind

caught her attention. Now she was not just being blown by the wind; she had become a part of it, blending and flowing with it in harmony. Because she made a choice, she has no need to rebel. Her energy can be used to move with the new direction instead of resisting it.

Because Louise is in a harmonious effort, the struggle in her mind is gone. She *prefers* what she has chosen to do. Each time she practices, she believes in her ability to choose, inner trust grows, and self-doubt wanes. With practice, she also believes more in her abilities to focus and guide her body and move her emotions to the center. With continued practice, she has more peak experiences, and she comes to value the practice more than reaching the peak. With the struggle turned into a preference and the finding of harmony in other new, self-chosen directions, her life transitions became smoother.

With each transition, life is less threatening. Inner security grows, and centeredness is increased, bringing out her best. In turn this builds her confidence, skills, insights, relationships, intellect, creativity, and general happiness as the conditions of her life (which she used to blame for her problems) continue to rise and fall without Louise falling apart (i.e., regaining her weight).

You can focus on and practice *mastery, empowerment,* and *wellness lifestyle* separately, and yet all lead to the same end. Each method blends into the other two at some point, and harmony will be attained by anyone who chooses to persist with any of the three. Individuals who achieve long-term success on their own most often use some parts or all of these methods of change.

How or if you define these methods is relatively unimportant compared to the personal desire to change. You have your own strength, purpose, and beliefs that will be directed where necessary as the need for adjustment in new situations arise. The method that you choose and own as yours is the one you will permit to work for you.

In the end the answers reside within you.

*   *   *

A Summary of Steps
To Personal Change

To see ourselves clearly, we must be calm and feel safe enough to be able to focus on what we have learned by observing, listening, and experiencing. To feel calm and safe over extended periods of time we must believe we can trust ourselves to get up and try again after we have fallen (risk taking) in our efforts to learn and grow. The follow-through practicing of mastery, the understanding and living out of a wellness lifestyle, and the consistency of empowerment behaviors will all lead to the intrinsic motivation required for long-term successful, balanced weight that requires effort but little or no mental struggle or conflict called procrastination.

The following summary of steps to personal change will help you start to create a new you. Learn them well enough to recall them as you need them each day.

The pounds on the scale and the number of calories don't determine long-term success with personal changes. Rather, it is the behavior and thinking that change self-image and the belief in the self that makes a difference in the final outcome. Several factors help people change their behavior, thoughts, and emotions.

- Know your beliefs (philosophy of life — what is true for you) that influence all behavior, thought, and emotion.
- Be clear as to your value priorities. Take a long look at what is important and how you live out your values from day to day. Does what you say you value match the way you spend your time?
- Nurture your self-worth by giving yourself equal caring time, energy, and thought as you do to meeting expectations, pleasing, and proving yourself by performance to others in your life.
- Learn intrinsic motivation by moving your focus off external motivations and goal orientations.
- Keep expectations modified, progressing at a moderate rate of change.

- Become familiar with your perfectionistic thoughts or behavior and modify them.
- Develop a healthy support group of friends and family that are positive models and can listen without taking control, parenting, or sabotaging your efforts.
- Safely make an educated change to healthful exercise for your energy, stimulation, and lifting depression with variety and balance.
- Become educated and comfortable with a regular, active healthful sexuality.
- Practice resolving your fears by slowly desensitizing yourself through your own initiation, confronting, embracing your fears, and staying close to the edge of your comfort zone.
- Learn to balance your wellness lifestyle with work-play, mental-physical activity, togetherness, and aloneness.
- Own your emotions by monitoring them and modifying your self-talk and mental images.
- Seek harmony over control by not defending the person you are, your values, or beliefs.
- Tune in to your intuition to be more spontaneous and less structured.
- Let go of self-criticalness in favor of self-affirmation and self-empowerment.
- Practice to reach mastery of a relaxation skill until you love the practice more than the outcome. Patience will be part of the secondary reward.
- Let go of how you were; refocus on the now and the evolving best you. The experience of the moment determines who you are becoming.
- Gradually change to healthful eating by taste preference emphasizing complex carbohydrates.

Once you've overcome the interal blocks that keep you from starting, everything in your life, including eating and exercise, will be in healthy harmony with your beliefs.

APPENDIX

Three-Phase Transitional Menu

I n keeping with the philosophical theme of this book, I don't offer the following three-phase menu as a weight-loss diet. It is only an *example* of how you may progressively choose a more healthful way to eat.

This sample menu is not meant to be your menu. But it will give you an awareness of the kind of menus you can create for yourself. You are most apt to stay with a menu created by you. This same thinking applies to recipes. You need to research and adapt recipes as you see fit. There are many resources available, some of which I have listed in the Bibliography.

When you create your own menu and recipes, you are proud of your ownership, and you are more likely to stick with it because you have created the recipes to suit your needs. Thus you remember them better and can prepare them more quickly. But most of all, you are in charge, not controlled by others.

As you mix healthful items more frequently into your menu, they will gradually dominate what you eat and even become your preferred choices. Even old fattening foods can be changed to healthful choices simply by adjusting them. Pizza, for example, can be made with a whole grain crust, vegetables instead of meat, and no-fat soy cheese.

Eat your new food choices routinely (without judgment or expectation) until you have psychologically come to accept them. The more you eat the new foods, or the new ingredients in old foods, the more your taste buds will appreciate them.

New healthful taste preferences are your long-term goal. If your changes are gradual and you do not mentally resist or push yourself, they will become preferred.

In each phase of your menu, keep in mind that you should be *avoiding* fats, excess protein, refined flours, sweeteners, and salt. At the same time you should be *increasing* your intake of fiber and carbohydrates. Choose whole grains whenever possible. Begin using whole fruit as your sweetener instead of sugars and artificial sweeteners. Reduce protein and turn to carbohydrates instead.

Several magazines, including *Vegetarian Times*, can offer you wonderful recipes that will help you with your change in food preferences. (They can also let you keep up-to-date on developments in nutrition and health.)

Choose from the menu items for each of the daily meals. Interchange new items with your usual foods as you move through the phases. The new foods of your choosing, such as those listed in Phase I, can be used in Phase II. And Phase II items can be used in Phase III to help you make that transition.

Plan to devote between three to six months for the entire three-phase transition. But don't feel that you should rush to keep a schedule. Nor should you stay in one phase if you think you are ready for the next.

Open up to new food choices by simply accepting them with greater regularity, keeping your self-talk as neutral as possible. Your taste buds will do the changing if your old biases are out of your mind. It isn't necessary to talk yourself into or out of these changes. Just practice and permit them. Progress begins as resistance ends.

PHASE I

Breakfast Menu

Egg substitute and chives
Whole grain breakfast food
Fresh fruit
Whole grain toast
Unsweetened applesauce
Non-fat milk or herb tea

Lunch Menu

Veggie (non-meat) burger
Whole grain burger bun
Large mixed vegetable salad
Basic vinaigrette dressing
Fresh fruit and fruit-sweetened cookie
Herb tea or mineral water

Dinner Menu

Broiled salmon filet
Broccoli
Non-fat cheese
Baked potato
Vegetable salad
Fresh fruit
Herb tea or mineral water

PHASE II

Breakfast Menu

Multigrain pancakes
Pureed pineapple topping (hot or cold)
Fresh melon
Herb tea

Lunch Menu

Broiled falafel
Whole grain pita pocket
Vegetable salad
Fruit and yogurt
Mineral water with ice

Dinner

Vegetable stew
Whole grain rye bread
Garden salad
Fresh fruit dipped in melted carob
Ice water and mint or herb tea

PHASE III

Breakfast

Multigrain hot cereal
    cooked in unfiltered apple juice with bananas
No-fat soy milk (on cereal)
Fresh fruit
Herb tea or hot carob and no-fat soy milk

Lunch

Vegetarian chili
Rice cakes with pureed fresh fruit
Non-dairy frozen dessert
Flavored mineral water with ice

Dinner

Baked lentil rice loaf
Steamed fresh or frozen peas
Vegetarian brown gravy
Mixed vegetable salad
Baked apple
Mineral water or herb tea

BIBLIOGRAPHY

The following publications have helped me develop my point of view toward weight loss through wellness. This is by no means a comprehensive list of all material available to you on the subject. Since the core of my attitude is that you must develop and manage your own program, I encourage you to discover additional resources that will help guide you.

Books

Altman, N. *Total Vegetarian Cooking*. New Canaan, CN: Keats Publishing Inc., 1981.

Ardell, Donald B., and John G. Langdon, M.D. *Wellness: The Body, Mind, and Spirit*. Dubuque: Kendall/Hunt Publishing Co., 1989.

Atrens, Dale M. *Don't Diet*. New York: William Morrow and Co., Inc., 1988.

Ballentine, R. *Transition To Vegetarianism*. Honesdale, PA: Himalayan Publishers, 1987.

Beck, Deva, and James Beck. *The Pleasure Connection*. San Marcos, CA: Synthesis Press, 1987.

Branden, Nathaniel. *Breaking Free*. New York: Bantam Books, Inc., 1987.

Branden, Nathaniel. *How To Raise Your Self-Esteem*. New York: Bantam Books, Inc. 1987.

Branden, Nathaniel. *The Power of Self-Esteem*. Deerfield, FL: Health Communications, Inc., 1992.

Bridges, William. *Transitions — Making Sense of Life's Changes*. Reading, MA: Addison-Wesley Publishing Co., 1980.

Broysenko, Joan. *Minding The Body, Mending The Mind*. New York: Bantam Books, Inc., 1987.

Bruno, F. J. *Think Yourself Thin*. New York: Barnes & Noble Books, 1972.

Bugental, James F. T. *Challenges Of Humanistic Psychology*. New York: McGraw-Hill Book Co., 1967.

Burka, J. B., and L. M. Yuen. *Procrastination: Why You Do It, What To Do About It*. Reading, MA: Addison-Wesley Publishing Co., 1983.

Chopra, Deepak. *Ageless Body, Timeless Mind*. New York: Harmony Books, 1993.

Crum, Thomas F. *The Magic of Conflict*. New York: Simon & Schuster, Inc., 1987.

Ellis, Albert, Michael Abrams, and Lidia Dengelegi. *The Art & Science of Rational Eating*. Fort Lee, NJ: Barricade Books Inc., 1992.

Ellis, Albert. *Reason and Emotion in Psychotherapy*. Secaucus, NJ: Citadel Press., 1962.

Fabry, Joseph. *Guideposts To Meaning*. Oakland: New Harbinger Publications, 1988.

Fanning, Patrick. *Visualization For Change*. Oakland: New Harbinger Publications, 1988.

Finando, S. J., and S. Mills. *Alternatives In Healing*. New York: NAL Books., 1989.

Frankl, Victor. *Man's Search For Meaning*. New York: Simon & Schuster, Inc., 1962.

Gershon, David, and Gail Straub. *Empowerment*. New York: Delta Books, 1989.

Goulart, F. S. *The Vegetarian Weightloss Cookbook*. New York: Simon & Schuster, Inc., 1982.

Hadley, Josie, and Carol Staudacher. *Hypnosis For Change*. Oakland: New Harbinger Publications, 1989.

Harman, Willis, and Howard Rheingold. *Higher Creativity — Liberating The Unconscious For Breakthrough Insights*. New York: Jeremy P. Tarcher, Inc., 1984.

Harp, D. *The Three Minute Meditator*. San Francisco: Mind's I Press, 1987.

Horowitz, Mardi, Charles Marmar, Janice Krupnick, Nancy Wilner, Nancy Kaltreider, Robert Wallerstein. *Personality Styles and Brief Psychotherapy*. New York: Basic Books, Inc., Publishers, 1984.

Hutchinson, M. G. *Transforming Body Image*. Freedom, CA: The Crossing Press, 1985.

Ilardo, Joseph. *Risk-Taking for Personal Growth*. Oakland: New Harbinger Publications. 1992.

Jampolsky, G. G. *Good-Bye To Guilt*. New York: Bantam Books, Inc. 1985.

Jeffers, Susan. *Feel The Fear And Do It Anyway*. New York: Ballantine Books, 1987.

Johnston, W. W. *Take Charge — A Guide To Feeling Good*. Gresham, OR: Acorn Endeavors, 1987.

Junshi, Chen, T. Colin Campbell, Li Junyao, and Richard Peto. *Diet, Life-style, and Mortality in China: A Study of the Characteristics of 65 Chinese Counties*. New York: Oxford University Press, 1990.

Kohn, Alfie. *No Contest: The Case Against Competition*. Boston: Houghton Mifflin, 1986.

Kopp, Sheldon B. *If You Meet The Buddha On The Road, Kill Him!* New York: Bantam Books, Inc., 1979.

Lad, V., M.D. *Ayurveda: "The Science Of Self-Healing"*. Santa Fe: Lotus Press, 1985.

Lazarus, A. *In The Mind's Eye*. New York: Guilford Press, 1984.

Leneman, L. *Slimming The Vegetarian Way*. Wellingborough, England: Thorsons Publishing, Ltd., 1989.

Leonard, George B. *The Transformation*. Los Angeles: J. P. Tarcher Inc., 1972.

Leonard, George. *Mastery*. New York: Penguin Books USA Inc., 1991.

Lowen, Alexander, M.D. *Fear of Life*. London: Collier MacMillan Publishers, 1980.

Ludeman, Kate. *The Worth Ethic*. New York: E.P. Dutton, 1989.

Maslow, Abraham H. *Motivation and Personality*. New York: Harper & Row, Publishers, Inc., 1970.

McClelland, David C. *Human Motivation*. Glenview, IL: Scott, Foresman and Company, 1985.

McClernan, James M. *Change Your Mind/Change Your Weight*. Sherwood, OR: Health Plus Publishers, 1985.
(P.O. Box 1027, Sherwood, OR. 97140 – 503-625-0589)

McDougall, John A., and Mary A. McDougall. *The McDougall Plan*. Piscataway, NJ: New Century Publishers, Inc., 1983.

McDougall, John A., M.D. *McDougall's Medicine*. Piscataway, NJ: New Century Publishers, Inc., 1985.

McDougall, Mary. *McDougall's Health Supportive Cookbook, Volume I.* Piscataway, NJ: New Century Publishers, Inc., 1985.

McDougall, Mary. *McDougall's Health Supportive Cookbook, Volume II.* Piscataway, NJ: New Century Publishers, Inc., 1986.

McKay, Matthew, and Patrick Fanning. *Prisoners of Belief.* Oakland: New Harbinger Publications, 1991.

McKay, Matthew, and Patrick Fanning. *Self-Esteem.* Oakland: New Harbinger Publications, 1987.

McMullin, R. E. *Handbook Of Cognitive Therapy Techniques.* New York: W.W. Norton and Co., 1986.

Meadow, Rosalyn, and Hillie Weiss. *Conflicts About Eating and Sexuality.* Binghampton, NY: Haworth Press, 1992.

Nader, Ralph. *Eating Clean.* Washington, D.C.: Center For Study of Responsive Law, 1982.

Nicholas, Mary W. *Change In The Context Of Group Therapy.* New York: Brunner/Mazel, Publishers, 1984.

Nozick, Robert. *The Examined Life.* New York: Simon & Schuster Inc., 1989.

Ornstein, Robert, and David Sobel, M.D. *The Healing Brain.* New York: Simon & Schuster, Inc., 1987.

Peele, Stanton. *Diseasing Of America — Addiction Treatment Out Of Control.* Lexington, MA: Lexington Books, 1989.

Peele, Stanton. *Love and Addiction.* New York: Taplinger Publishing Co., 1975.

Read, R., M.D., and T. Rusk, M.D. *I Want To Change — But I Don't Know How!* Los Angeles: Price/Stern/Sloan, 1986.

Robbins, John. *Diet For A New America.* Walpole, NH: Stillpoint Publishing, 1987.

Rossi, Ernest Lawrence. *The Psychobiology Of Mind-Body Healing.* New York: W. W. Norton and Co. Inc., 1986.

Rossman, M. L. *Healing Yourself.* New York: Walker and Co., 1987.

Rubin, Theodore I., M.D. *Overcoming Indecisiveness.* New York: Harper and Row Publishers, 1985.

Satala, C. *Awaken Your Creative Potential.* Fort Wayne, IN: CLS Press, 1988.

Selby, A. *Procrastinator's Success Kit*. Portland, OR: Beynch Press, 1986

Siroka, Robert W., Ellen K. Siroka, and Gilbert A. Schloss. *Sensitivity Training and Group Encounter*. New York: Grosset & Dunlap, 1971.

Slochower, J. A. *Excessive Eating: The Role Of Emotions and Environment*. New York: Human Sciences Press, 1983.

Stock, Gregory. *The Book of Questions*. New York: Workman Publishing Co., 1987.

Tart, Charles T. *Waking Up — Overcoming The Obstacles To Human Potential*. Boston: New Science Library, 1986.

Thrash, Agatha, M.D. *Eat For Strength — A Vegetarian Cookbook*. Lillington, NC: Edwards Brothers, Inc., 1978.

Tracy, Lisa. *The Gradual Vegetarian*. New York: Dell Publishers, 1985.

Trimpey, Jack. *The Small Book*. New York: Delacorte Press, 1992.

Vickery, Donald M., M.D. and James F. Fries, M.D. *Take Care of Yourself — The Consumer's Guide to Medical Care*. Reading, MA: Addison-Wesley Publishing Co., 1986.

Von Oech, Roger D. *A Kick In The Seat Of The Pants*. New York: Perennial Library, 1986.

Von Oech, Roger D. *A Whack On The Side Of The Head*. New York: Warner Books, 1983.

Watts, Alan W. *The Wisdom Of Insecurity*. New York: Vintage Books, 1951.

Weil, Andrew, M.D., and W. Rosen. *Chocolate To Morphine*. Boston: Houghton Mifflin Co., 1983.

Weiner, M. A. *Maximum Immunity*. Boston: Houghton Mifflin Co., 1986.

Woitita, Janet G. *Struggle For Intimacy*. Deerfield Beach, FL: Health Communications, Inc., 1985.

Wolpe, Joseph, M.D. *Life Without Fear — Anxiety and Its Cure*. Oakland: New Harbinger Publications, 1988.

Wurtman, J. J. *Managing Your Mind And Mood Through Food*. New York: Rawson Associates, 1986.

Periodicals

"Consumers Guide To Low Fat Shopping." *Prevention* (January 1991): 75-134.

"Cutting The Fat." *Vegetarian Times* (April, 1991).

"Green Seal." *Delicious Magazine* (November/December 1990): 4.

"Losing Weight: What Works, What Doesn't." *Consumer Reports* (June 1993): 347-357.

"Oprah Mum On Any Weight Gain." *Tufts University Diet and Nutrition Letter, Special Report* (February 1990).

"Organic Outlook." *Delicious Magazine* (October 1990): 43.

"The End Of The Diet Boom...and Bust." *American Health Magazine* (January/February 1990): 120.

"Yo-Yo Dieting Increases Heart Attack Rates." *Arizona Republic* (January 17, 1993): A3.

Beck, Melinda, Karen Springen, Lucille Beachy, Mary Hager, and Linda Buckley. "The Losing Formula." *Newsweek* (April 30, 1990): 52.

Blakeslee, Sandra. "New Connections." *American Health Magazine* (March 1990): 74.

Bray, George A., and David S. Gray. "Obesity Part II — Treatment." *Western Journal of Medicine* (November 1988): 555-571.

Campbell, Colin T. "The Study On Diet, Nutrition and Disease In The People's Republic Of China." *Contemporary Nutrition 14* (1989): 6.

Elleson, Vera J. "Competition: A Cultural Imperative." *The Personnel And Guidance Journal* (December 1983): 195-198.

Fatis, Michael, Alane Weiner, JoAnn Hawkins, and Brent Van Dorsten. "Following Up On A Commercial Weight-Loss Program: Do The Pounds Stay Off After Your Picture Has Been In The Newspaper?" *Journal Of The American Dietetic Association* 89 no. 4 (April 1989).

Ferguson, Tom, M.D. "The Anatomy Of Empowerment." *Medical Self-Care Magazine* (January/February 1989): 72.

Fletcher, Anne M. "The Yo-Yo Enzyme." *American Health Magazine* (October 1990): 85.

Friedman, Richard B., M.D. "Very Low Calorie Diets: How Successful?" *Postgraduate Medicine*, vol. 83 no. 6 (May 1, 1988).

Gallagher, Winifred, and Joel Gurin. "Change." *American Health
Magazine* (March 1990): 49-52.

Grilow, Carlos M., Saul Shiffman, and Rena R. Wing. "Relapse Crises
and Coping Among Dieters." *Journal of Consulting & Clinical
Psychology*, vol. 57, no. 4 (1989): 488-499.

Gurin, Joel. "Eating Goes Back To Basics." *American Health Magazine*
(March 1990): 96.

Gurin, Joel, "Leaner, Not Lighter." *Psychology Today*. (March 1989):
32-36.

Hovell, Melbourne F., Alma Koch, C. Richard Hofstetter, Carol Sipan,
Patricia Faucher, Ann Dellinger, Gerald Borok, Alan Forsythe,
and Vincent J. Felitti, M.D. "Long-Term Weight Loss Maintenance: Assessment of a Behavioral and Supplemented Fasting
Regimen." *American Journal of Public Health*, vol. 78, no. 6 (June
1988).

Kirschner, Marvin A., George Schneider, Norman H. Ertel, and Joan
Gorman. "An Eight-Year Experience With A Very-Low-Calorie
Formula Diet For Control Of Major Obesity." *International Jour-
nal of Obesity* 12 (July 1987): 69-80.

Kohn, Alfie. "The Case Against Competition." *Noetic Sciences Review*
(Spring 1990): 12-19.

Kramer, Matthew F., Robert W. Jeffery, Jean L. Forster, and Mary
Kaye Snell. "Long-Term Follow-Up of Behavioral Treatment For
Obesity: Patterns of Weight Regain Among Men and Women."
International Journal of Obesity 13 (1989): 123-136.

Krizmanic, Judy. "What's In A Label." *Vegetarian Times* (July 1989):
27-33.

Lavery, Margaret A., John W. Loewy, Asha S. Kapadia, Milton Z.
Nichaman, M.D., John P. Foreyt, and Molly Gee. "Long-Term
Follow-Up Of Weight Status Of Subjects In A Behavioral Weight
Control Program." *Journal Of The American Dietetic Association*
89 (1989): 1259-1264.

Lefebvre, Craig R., Elizabeth A. Harden, William Rakowski, Thomas
M. Lasater, and Richard A. Carleton, M.D. "Characteristics Of
Participants In Community Health Promotion Programs: Four-

Year Results." *American Journal Of Public Health* vol. 77, no. 10 (October 1987).

Liddle, R.A., R. B. Goldstein, and J. Saxton. "Gallstone Formation During Weight-Reduction Dieting." *Archives of Internal Medicine* vol. 148, no. 8 (August 1989): 1750-3.

MacLean, Lloyd D., M.D. "Surgery For Obesity: Where Do We Go From Here?" *American College Of Surgeons Bulletin* vol. 74, no. 9, Spectrum (1989).

McClernan, James. "Take My Body Please." *Men's Fitness Magazine* (October 1987): 36.

McClernan, James. "The Magic Of Weight Control." *Health World Magazine* (Summer 1987): 11.

McClernan, James. "Hungry For Success." *SHAPE Magazine* vol. 6, no. 8 (April 1987): 102.

McClernan, James. "Ms. Perfect." *SHAPE Magazine* vol. 5, no. 8 (April 1986): 82.

McClernan, James. "Love Relationships." *SHAPE Magazine* vol. 5, no. 6 (February 1986).

McClernan, James. "You Can Defeat The Manana Syndrome." *SHAPE Magazine* vol. 4, no. 5 (January 1985).

Perri, Michael G., Arthur M. Nezu, Eugene T. Patti, and Karen L. McCann. "Effect Of Length Of Treatment On Weight Loss." *Journal Of Consulting and Clinical Psychology* vol. 57, no. 3 (1989): 450-452.

Peterson, Francis J. "Summary Of The Sophos and The Optifast Core Program Phase 1 Clinical Trials and The Sandoz Nutrition Collaborative Study Group A, B." Sandoz Nutrition Corporation (1987).

Ravussin, Eric, and Clifton Bogardus, M.D. "Relationship of Genetics, Age, and Physical Fitness To Daily Energy Expenditure and Fuel Utilization." *American Journal of Clinical Nutrition* 49 (1989): 968.

Ravussin, Eric, Stephen Lillioja, William C. Knowler, M.D., Laurent Christin, M.D., Daniel Freymond, M.D., William G. H. Abbott, M.D., Vicky Boyce, Barbara V. Howard, and Clifton Bogardue, M.D. "Reduced Rate of Energy Expenditure As A Risk Factor For

Body-Weight Gain." *The New England Journal of Medicine* (February 25, 1988): 467-472.

Ravussin, Eric., Stephen Lillioja, Thomas E. Anderson, Laurent Christin, and Clifton Bogardus. "Determinants of 24-hour Energy Expenditure in Man." *The Journal of Clinical Investigation*, vol. 78 (December 1986): 1568-1578.

Rosenblatt, Elaine. "Weight-Loss Programs: Pluses and Minuses of Commercial and Self-Help Groups." *Postgraduate Medicine*, vol 83, no 6 (May 1, 1988).

Rubin, Rita, Densie Webb, David Schardt, Carl Lowe, and Kim C. Flodin. "Lose Weight and Keep It Off!" *American Health Magazine Special Report* (July/August 1991): 45.

Sauer, Jennings Cheryl. "What Have You Got To Lose?" *American Health Magazine* (March, 1989): 155.

Seaton, Timothy B., M.D., Steve Heymsfield, M.D., and William Rosenthal, M.D. "Ursodeoxycholic Acid and Gallstones During Weight Loss." *The New England Journal Of Medicine* vol. 320, no. 20 (May 18, 1989): 1351.

Sikand, Geeta, Albert Kondo, John P. Foreyt, Peter H. Jones, M.D., and Antonio M. Gotto, Jr. M.D. "Two-Year Follow-Up of Patients Treated With A Very-Low-Calorie Diet and Exercise Training." *Journal of The American Dietetic Association* vol. 88, no. 4 (April 1988): 487.

Tessler, Gordon. "Lose Weight Without Counting Calories." *Total Health Magazine* (October 1989): 15.

Wadden, Thomas A., Albert J. Stunkard, M.D., and Jane Liebschutz, M.D. "Three-Year Follow-Up Of The Treatment Of Obesity by Very Low Calorie Diet, Behavior Therapy, and Their Combination." *Journal of Consulting and Clinical Psychology* vol. 56, no. 6 (1988): 925-928.

Wadden, Thomas A., Theodore B. Van Itallie, M.D., and George L. Blackburn, M.D. "Responsible and Irresponsible Use Of Very-Low-Calorie Diets In Treatment Of Obesity." *Journal of American Medical Association* vol. 263, no. 1 (January 5, 1990).

Young, Eleanor A., Rodolfo G. Ramos, and Merle M. Harris. "Gastrointestinal and Cardiac Response To Low-Calorie Semistarvation Diets." *American Journal of Clinical Nurtrition* 47 (1988): 981-988.

About the Author

Dr. James McClernan has been treating individuals suffering from addictions, including the addiction to food, for more than 20 years.

As a licensed psychologist, he has practiced in hospital, corporate, university, military, and private settings. His experience includes proficiency in numerous modalities ranging from existential psychotherapy and aversion conditioning to biofeedback and gestalt groups. He has also taught at four state universities, conducted research for a Fortune 500 company, been a presenter at conferences and seminars, and conducts his own wellness workshops. Dr. McClernan is a past Regional Coordinator for seven states and British Columbia of the Association for Humanistic Psychology. He also conducts a private psychotherapy practice.

In addition to *Hugs from the Refrigerator*, Dr. McClernan has written *Change Your Mind/Change Your Weight* (Health Plus Publishers, 1985) and over 40 articles for magazines and journals. He has appeared on more than 100 radio and television programs in the United States, Canada, and Australia.